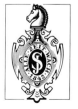

R. Nieuwenhuys   J. Voogd
Chr. van Huijzen

The Human
Central Nervous System

A Synopsis and Atlas

Second Revised Edition

With 154 Figures

Springer-Verlag
Berlin Heidelberg New York 1981

RUDOLF NIEUWENHUYS, M.D.
Professor of Neuroanatomy, Department of Anatomy,
University of Nijmegen, The Netherlands

JAN VOOGD, M.D.
Professor of Neuroanatomy, Department of Anatomy,
University of Leiden, The Netherlands and
Department of Anatomy, Free University of Brussels (V.U.B.),
Belgium

CHRISTIAAN VAN HUIJZEN
Medical artist, Department of Anatomy, University of Nijmegen,
The Netherlands

ISBN 3-540-10316-3 2. Auflage Springer-Verlag Berlin Heidelberg New York
ISBN 0-387-10316-3 2nd Edition Springer-Verlag New York Heidelberg Berlin

ISBN 3-540-08903-9 1. Auflage Springer-Verlag Berlin Heidelberg New York
ISBN 0-387-08903-9 1st Edition Springer-Verlag New York Heidelberg Berlin

Library of Congress Cataloging in Publication Data. NIEUWENHUYS, R. 1927–   . The human central nervous system. Bibliography: p.   . Includes index. 1. Central nervous system-Atlases. 2. Histology-Atlases. 3. Neuroanatomy-Atlases. I. VOOGD, J., joint author. II. HUIJZEN, CHR. VAN, joint author. III. Title. [DNLM: 1. Central nervous system-Anatomy and histology-Atlases. WL17 N682h] QM455.N48 1980 612'.82'0222 80 –23070
Reproduction of figures: Gustav Dreher GmbH, Stuttgart
Typesetting, printing, and bookbinding by Universitätsdruckerei H. Stürtz AG, Würzburg
2121/3130-54321

Preface to the Second Edition

The particularly good reception enjoyed by our "The Human Central Nervous System, a Synopsis and Atlas" has made a second edition necessary, hardly more than two years after its first appearance. This new edition enabled us to make a number of corrections, but it was judged premature to undertake a thorough updating of the text. However, a major improvement — suggested by some reviewers and many colleagues — is that in this new edition the abbreviations in the figures have been replaced by the full Latin terms.

We want to emphasize that the study of this book can facilitate and deepen but never replace the study of the anatomical preparation. Acquaintance with the basic cytology and histology of nervous tissue has been taken for granted.

This book is evidently often consulted with the aim of looking up a particular structure together with its name and its topographical relations. This is certainly one of the purposes of the book. We are, however, of the opinion that during a systematic study of the figures showing the functional systems in part IV, perusal of the accompanying text will be necessary. As a matter of fact the spatial representations of the fibre systems are no more than a visualization of the most salient features discussed in the text. The pictures are so to speak a snapshot of the current knowledge of a particular functional system within the central nervous system; no less, but no more either. The mutual coherence between the pictures in the macroscopical, microscopical and functional sections of the book, will be readily apparent during the use of the work. The authors hope that for the readers this coherence will lead to a better insight into the structure of the human central nervous system.

Spring 1981   R. NIEUWENHUYS
                                                           J. VOOGD
                                                           CHR. VAN HUIJZEN

Contents

Introduction

Purpose and Plan

This atlas has been designed with the object of providing a comprehensive pictorial survey of the macroscopic and microscopic structure of the human central nervous system.

The pictorial material encompasses 154 half-tone and line drawings, all derived from original macroscopic and microscopic preparations. Considerable thought has been given in the preparation of these drawings to an optimal combination of clarity and exactness. Moreover great pains have been taken to achieve a maximal coherence of thematically related figures. The illustrations are arranged in four sections. The first section depicts the gross appearance and three-dimensional structure of the brain and spinal cord. The second section includes drawings of a number of whole brain slices, sectioned in four different directions. The third section consists of a carefully selected series of 25 microscopic sections through the spinal cord, brain stem and basal prosencephalon. In these sections the fibre systems are shown on the right and the cell masses on the left side. The final section integrates and amplifies the data presented in the preceding sections. The central nervous system is divided here into eleven functional systems and the interrelationships of the centres and fibre paths belonging to each of these systems are depicted and briefly described. Emphasis has been laid on aspects of clinical significance.

This atlas, though primarily intended for medical students, may also be expected to be useful as a quick pictorial review for practitioners in the various neurological sciences.

Material, Techniques, and Preparation of the Illustrations

The gross anatomical section of this atlas is based on eight brains and one spinal cord of adult individuals with no record of neurological diseases. These specimens were fixed for at least two months in formalin. One specimen was used for the illustrations showing the external morphology. This brain was then serially sliced into 2-mm-thick sections in the coronal plane. Three other brains were sliced in the three other conventional planes: sagittal, horizontal and perpendicular to the axis of the brain stem. The serial slices thus obtained were employed in the preparation of various graphical and three-dimensional reconstructions. The latter were made from 4-mm-thick styrofoam sheets. The remaining four brains were dissected in a number of ways. All of the figures in this section showing features of the internal configuration of the brain are based on reconstructions or dissections or both. Therefore, in these figures the size, shape and spatial relationships of the structures revealed are reproduced with great exactitude.

The brain slices that constitute the second section of this atlas were selected from the four series of slices already mentioned. The brains were embedded in gelatin and sliced on a rotary-blade commercial meat slicer. Due to the elasticity of the large gelatin blocks we experienced initially considerable difficulties in maintaining the intended plane of sectioning throughout a series. However, this problem was ingeniously solved by Mr. A. BINNENDIJK, our laboratory assistant, by embedding the brains in boxes, prepared from styrofoam plates, and by subsequently slicing the brains while still encased in the surrounding box. This procedure yielded perfect, well-oriented, continuous series of slices.

The microscopical sections that comprise the third section were all drawn from original preparations. The sections through the basal prosencephalon are based on one of the excellent Weigert-Pal series which the late Professor G. JELGERSMA employed for his Atlas Anatomicum Cerebri Humani [114] and on a series of Klüver-Barrera preparations. The procedure was as follows. Seven sections were selected from the Weigert-Pal series. From these sections outline drawings were prepared at a magnification of four diameters in which the position of the fibre systems and cell masses was indicated. Since the series only includes one half of the brain, the other half was added in the drawings as a mirror image. In order to obtain bilateral symmetry slight corrections appeared to be necessary. In the right half of the drawings the fibre pattern was drawn in semi-diagrammatically. The cell masses were studied in corresponding sections of the Klüver-Barrera series. From each griseum one or several characteristic samples were drawn at a magnification of 40 diameters with the aid of a projection apparatus. These samples were employed for depicting the cell masses in the left halves of the sections. Thus, it should be appreciated that the cells are represented

at a magnification ten times that of the section as a whole.

The sections through the brain stem and the spinal cord are based on Nissl and Häggqvist material. The latter technique was selected for the analysis of the white matter, because it shows both the axon and the myelin sheath of the individual nerve fibres in contrasting colours. Neuronal somata can also be observed in Häggqvist material, though with less distinctness than in Nissl sections. The procedure followed in the preparation of the drawings involved the following sequence of steps:

1) Häggqvist sections of the levels to be depicted were selected.

2) With the aid of a photographic enlarger negative photographic prints of these sections with a magnification of seven diameters were made.

3) Under microscopic control the various areas of grey and white matter were delineated on the photographs. In this way outline drawings for the final figures were obtained.

4) The fibre composition and the fibre pattern of the various tracts and more diffuse areas of white matter were analysed; the fibres were graded into three groups: coarse, medium or thin. By using dots and lines of corresponding diameters the results of the analysis were represented semi-diagrammatically in the drawings.

5) From corresponding Nissl preparations samples of the various nuclei and other cellular areas were drawn at a magnification of 70 diameters. These samples were employed for depicting the cell masses in the left halves of the drawings. Thus, in this series of drawings, as in those of the sections through the forebrain, the neuronal somata are represented at a magnification ten times that of the sections as a whole.

The pictures constituting the fourth and final section fall into two categories: (1)

plates showing the topographic relationships of the structures belonging to the various functional systems and (2) diagrams illustrating the neuronal interrelationships within these systems. The plates are largely based on reconstructions prepared from our own macroscopic and microscopic material. The diagrams are based on data compiled from the literature.

Annotations

An effort has been made to enhance the usefulness of this atlas by including brief descriptions of the functional systems depicted. These annotations include the most important findings of modern experimental neuroanatomical research.

Terminology and Labelling

Since the Latin terminology has the obvious advantage of accepted international usage, it was decided to employ this terminology wherever possible. However, to facilitate use of the atlas we have included the English or Anglicised equivalents wherever they seemed important in the index. As regards gross anatomy, the Paris Nomina Anatomica, which were adopted in 1955 by the International Nomenclature Committee and revised in 1960 and 1965, has been used. Unfortunately an internationally approved nomenclature for the microscopic structures of the brain does not exist. For the nomenclature of these structures various works have been consulted, among which the atlases of RILEY [216], SCHALTENBRAND and BAILEY [225], and SINGER and YAKOVLEV [232], should be especially mentioned. Our principal sources for interpretation and terminology of structures in partic-

ular brain regions were as follows: Cell masses of the brain stem: OLSZEWSKI and BAXTER [196]; cerebellum: ANGEVINE, et al. [8]; thalamus: DEWULF [63] and VAN BUREN and BORKE [257]; hypothalamus: NAUTA and HAYMAKER [183]; allocortical and adjacent structures: STEPHAN [235]; amygdala: CROSBY and HUMPHREY [50].

It was not feasible to label all of the recognisable structures on every plate. In the series of slices (Sect. II) and microscopical sections (Sect. III) structures that appear repeatedly have been labelled on alternative plates or, in a number of instances, even less frequently.

Acknowledgements

The generous support of the medical faculties of Nijmegen and Leiden is gratefully acknowledged.

The authors wish to thank Dr. J.H.R. SCHOEN for making available the Häggqvist material, Mr. A. BINNENDIJK and Mr. C. CORNELISSEN for the preparation of the series of brain slices and Mrs. C. de VOCHT-POORT, Miss P.N. VERIJDT and Mr. J. STINS for the preparation of the histological material.

Acknowledgement is made to the artists: to Mr. T. VAN GERWEN, who made the half-tone illustrations, to Mr. A. GRUTER, who did the drawings of the microscopical sections, and to Mr. W.P.J. MAAS, who prepared most of the line drawings and also aided in the labelling of the illustrations. Without their skill and patience this atlas would have been impossible.

We are deeply indebted to Dr. I.H.M. SMART for critically reading and checking the English of the manuscript.

The invaluable secretarial assistance of Mrs. G.E.J.M. VAN SON-VERSTRAETEN is especially acknowledged.

Finally, the authors extend their most sincere thanks to the publishing house of Springer and their co-workers — especially Mrs. TH. DEIGMÖLLER, Mrs. D. GROSS-HANS, Mr. E. ERFLING and Mrs. U. PFAFF for their continued help during the preparation and publication of this book.

Part I Gross Anatomy

Orientation

External and Medial Views

Internal Structures

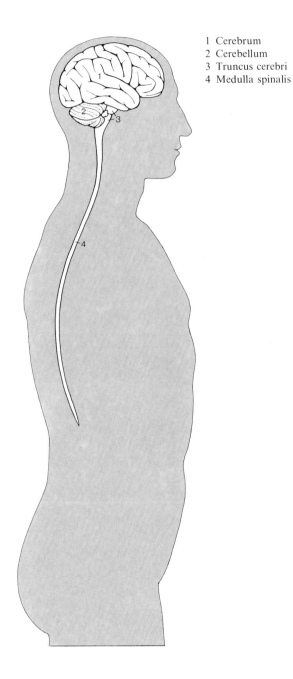

1 Cerebrum
2 Cerebellum
3 Truncus cerebri
4 Medulla spinalis

Fig. 1. The central nervous system in situ (1/6×)

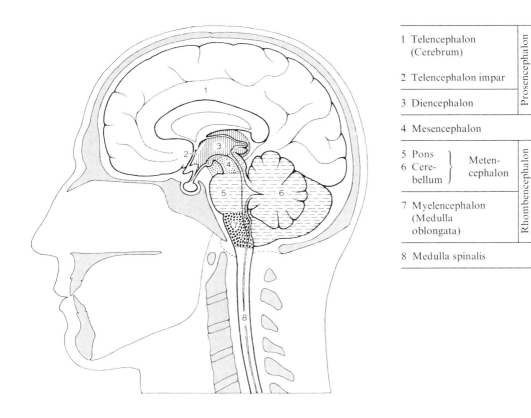

1 Telencephalon (Cerebrum)	Prosencephalon		Neuraxis (Systema nervosum centrale)
2 Telencephalon impar			
3 Diencephalon			
4 Mesencephalon		Truncus cerebri / Encephalon	
5 Pons 6 Cerebellum } Metencephalon	Rhombencephalon		
7 Myelencephalon (Medulla oblongata)			
8 Medulla spinalis			

Fig. 2. Medial surface of the right half of the brain in the bisected head. The position of its major subdivisions is indicated (2/5×)

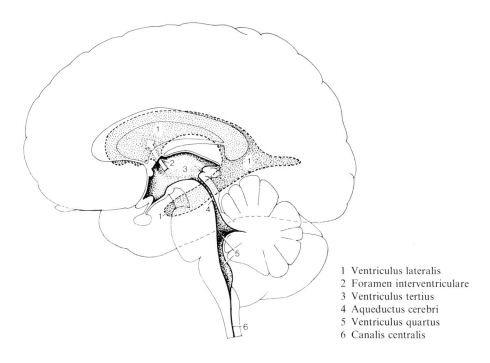

1 Ventriculus lateralis
2 Foramen interventriculare
3 Ventriculus tertius
4 Aqueductus cerebri
5 Ventriculus quartus
6 Canalis centralis

Fig. 3. The ventricular system of the brain. The *arrow* passes through the foramen interventriculare from the third ventricle to the lateral ventricle ($3/5 \times$)

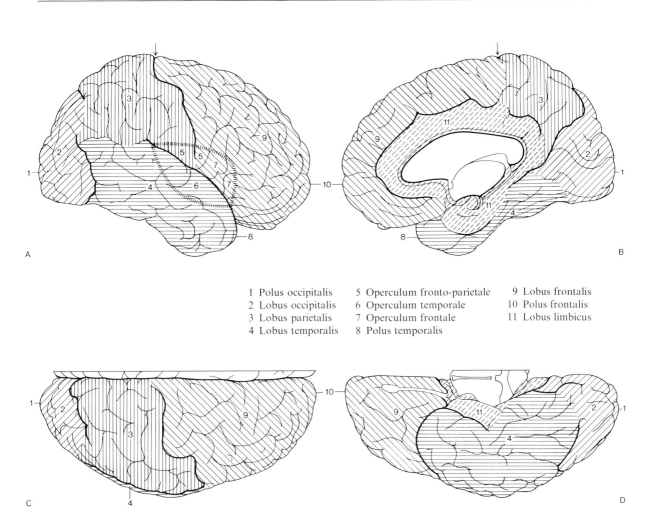

1 Polus occipitalis	5 Operculum fronto-parietale	9 Lobus frontalis
2 Lobus occipitalis	6 Operculum temporale	10 Polus frontalis
3 Lobus parietalis	7 Operculum frontale	11 Lobus limbicus
4 Lobus temporalis	8 Polus temporalis	

Fig. 4A–D. Subdivision of the right cerebral hemisphere into lobes. **A** lateral view; **B** medial view; **C** superior view; **D** inferior view (1/2 ×)

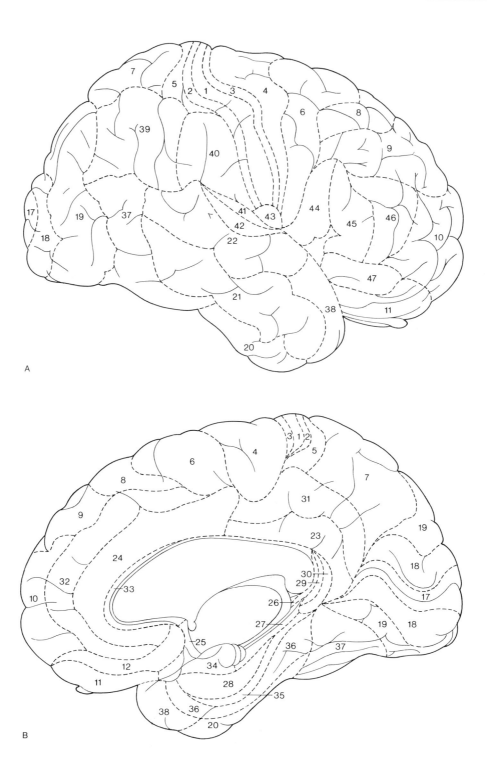

Fig. 5A and B. Subdivision of the cortex of the right cerebral hemisphere into cytoarchitectonic fields according to Brodmann (3/4 ×). **A** lateral view; **B** medial view

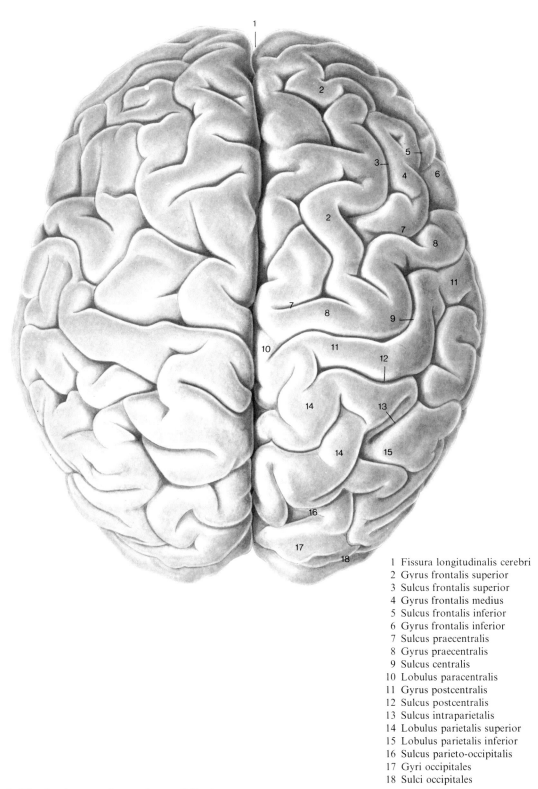

Fig. 6. The brain seen from above (1/1 ×)

1 Fissura longitudinalis cerebri
2 Gyrus frontalis superior
3 Sulcus frontalis superior
4 Gyrus frontalis medius
5 Sulcus frontalis inferior
6 Gyrus frontalis inferior
7 Sulcus praecentralis
8 Gyrus praecentralis
9 Sulcus centralis
10 Lobulus paracentralis
11 Gyrus postcentralis
12 Sulcus postcentralis
13 Sulcus intraparietalis
14 Lobulus parietalis superior
15 Lobulus parietalis inferior
16 Sulcus parieto-occipitalis
17 Gyri occipitales
18 Sulci occipitales

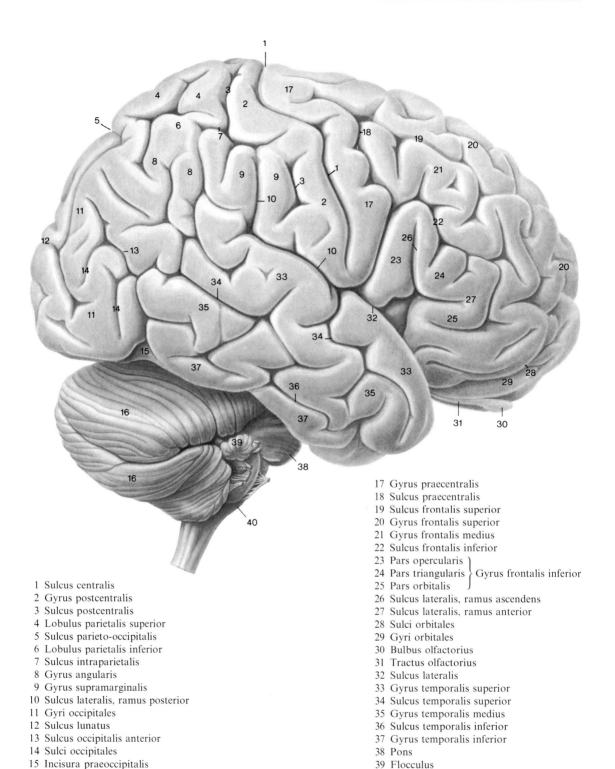

1 Sulcus centralis
2 Gyrus postcentralis
3 Sulcus postcentralis
4 Lobulus parietalis superior
5 Sulcus parieto-occipitalis
6 Lobulus parietalis inferior
7 Sulcus intraparietalis
8 Gyrus angularis
9 Gyrus supramarginalis
10 Sulcus lateralis, ramus posterior
11 Gyri occipitales
12 Sulcus lunatus
13 Sulcus occipitalis anterior
14 Sulci occipitales
15 Incisura praeoccipitalis
16 Hemisphaerium cerebelli

17 Gyrus praecentralis
18 Sulcus praecentralis
19 Sulcus frontalis superior
20 Gyrus frontalis superior
21 Gyrus frontalis medius
22 Sulcus frontalis inferior
23 Pars opercularis ⎫
24 Pars triangularis ⎬ Gyrus frontalis inferior
25 Pars orbitalis ⎭
26 Sulcus lateralis, ramus ascendens
27 Sulcus lateralis, ramus anterior
28 Sulci orbitales
29 Gyri orbitales
30 Bulbus olfactorius
31 Tractus olfactorius
32 Sulcus lateralis
33 Gyrus temporalis superior
34 Sulcus temporalis superior
35 Gyrus temporalis medius
36 Sulcus temporalis inferior
37 Gyrus temporalis inferior
38 Pons
39 Flocculus
40 Medulla oblongata

Fig. 7. Lateral view of the brain (1/1 ×)

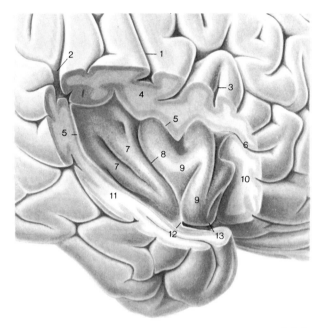

1 Sulcus centralis
2 Sulcus lateralis, ramus posterior
3 Sulcus lateralis, ramus ascendens
4 Operculum fronto-parietale
5 Sulcus circularis insulae
6 Sulcus lateralis, ramus anterior
7 Gyrus longus insulae
8 Sulcus centralis insulae
9 Gyri breves insulae
10 Operculum frontale
11 Operculum temporale
12 Limen insulae
13 Polus insulae

Fig. 8. Dissection of the right cerebral hemisphere to display the insula (1/1 ×)

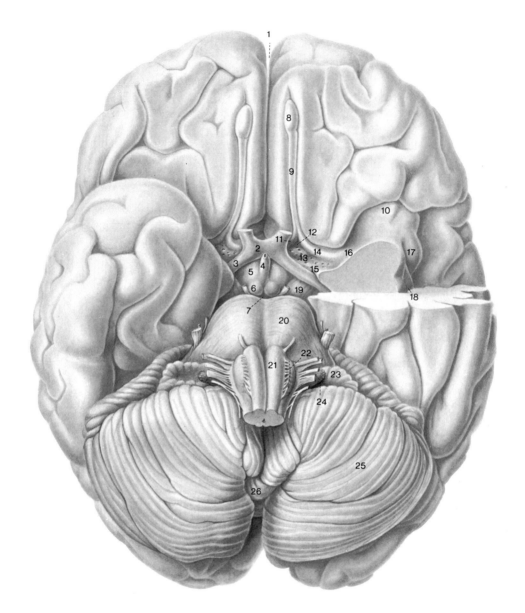

1 Fissura longitudinalis cerebri
2 Chiasma opticum
3 Tractus opticus
4 Infundibulum
5 Tuber cinereum
6 Corpus mamillare
7 Fossa interpeduncularis

8 Bulbus olfactorius
9 Tractus olfactorius
10 Polus insulae
11 Stria olfactoria medialis
12 Trigonum olfactorium
13 Substantia perforata anterior
14 Stria olfactoria lateralis
15 Gyrus diagonalis
16 Limen insulae
17 Gyri breves insulae

18 Gyrus longus insulae
19 Pedunculus cerebri
20 Pons
21 Pyramis
22 Oliva
23 Flocculus
24 Plexus choroideus ventriculi
   quarti
25 Hemisphaerium cerebelli
26 Vermis cerebelli

Fig. 9. Basal view of the brain. The frontal portion of the left temporal lobe has been removed to expose the underlying structures (1/1 ×)

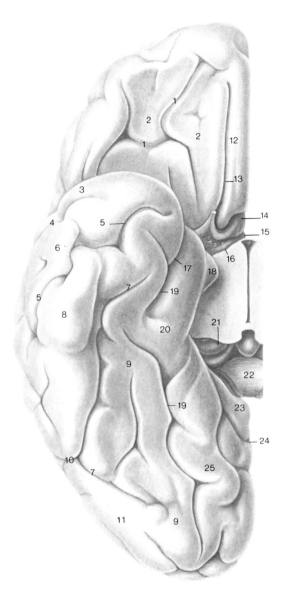

1 Sulci orbitales
2 Gyri orbitales
3 Gyrus temporalis superior
4 Sulcus temporalis superior
5 Sulcus temporalis inferior
6 Gyrus temporalis medius
7 Sulcus occipitotemporalis
8 Gyrus temporalis inferior
9 Gyrus occipitotemporalis
   lateralis
10 Incisura praeoccipitalis
11 Gyri occipitales

12 Gyrus rectus
13 Sulcus olfactorius
14 Area subcallosa
15 Gyrus paraterminalis
16 Gyrus diagonalis
17 Sulcus rhinalis
18 Gyrus ambiens
19 Sulcus collateralis
20 Gyrus parahippocampalis
21 Pulvinar thalami
22 Splenium corporis callosi
23 Isthmus gyri cinguli
24 Sulcus calcarinus
25 Gyrus occipitotemporalis
   medialis

Fig. 10. Basal view of the right cerebral hemisphere. The olfactory tract has been sectioned (1/1 ×)

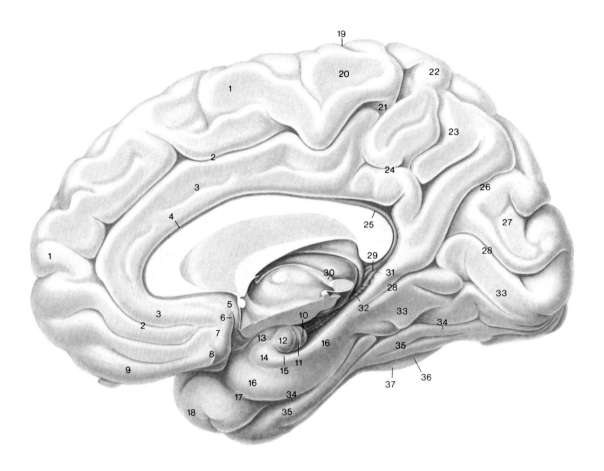

1 Gyrus frontalis superior
2 Sulcus cinguli
3 Gyrus cinguli
4 Sulcus corporis callosi
5 Gyrus paraterminalis
6 Sulcus parolfactorius posterior
7 Area subcallosa
8 Sulcus parolfactorius anterior
9 Gyrus rectus
10 Gyrus intralimbicus ⎫
11 Limbus Giacomini ⎬ Uncus
12 Gyrus uncinatus ⎭
13 Gyrus semilunaris
14 Gyrus ambiens
15 Incisura unci
16 Gyrus parahippocampalis
17 Sulcus rhinalis
18 Gyrus temporalis superior

19 Sulcus centralis
20 Lobulus paracentralis
21 Sulcus cinguli, pars marginalis
22 Lobulus parietalis superior
23 Praecuneus
24 Sulcus subparietalis
25 Indusium griseum
26 Sulcus parieto-occipitalis
27 Cuneus
28 Sulcus calcarinus
29 Gyrus fasciolaris
30 Taenia thalami
31 Isthmus gyri cinguli
32 Gyrus dentatus
33 Gyrus occipitotemporalis medialis
34 Sulcus collateralis
35 Gyrus occipitotemporalis lateralis
36 Sulcus occipitotemporalis
37 Gyrus temporalis inferior

Fig. 11. Medial aspect of the right cerebral hemisphere (1/1 ×)

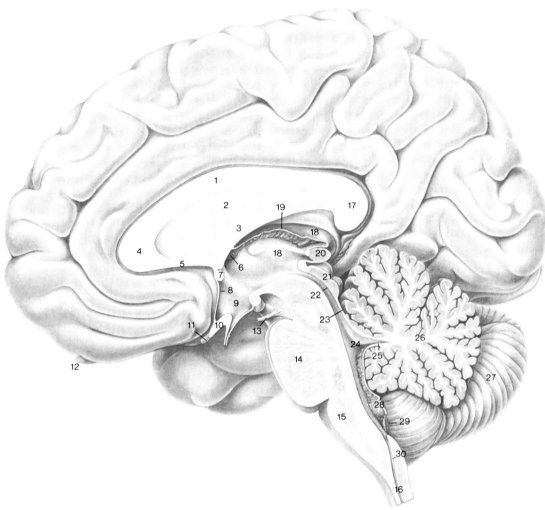

1 Truncus corporis callosi
2 Septum pellucidum
3 Fornix
4 Genu corporis callosi
5 Rostrum corporis callosi
6 Foramen interventriculare
7 Commissura anterior
8 Lamina terminalis
9 Hypothalamus
10 Chiasma opticum
11 Nervus opticus
12 Bulbus olfactorius
13 Nervus oculomotorius
14 Pons
15 Medulla oblongata
16 Medulla spinalis

17 Splenium corporis callosi
18 Thalamus
19 Tela choroidea ventriculi tertii
20 Corpus pineale
21 Lamina quadrigemina
22 Aqueductus cerebri
23 Velum medullare superius
24 Ventriculus quartus
25 Velum medullare inferius
26 Vermis cerebelli
27 Hemisphaerium cerebelli
28 Tela choroidea ventriculi quarti
29 Apertura mediana ventriculi quarti
30 Canalis centralis

Fig. 12. Medial view of the right half of the bisected brain (1/1×)

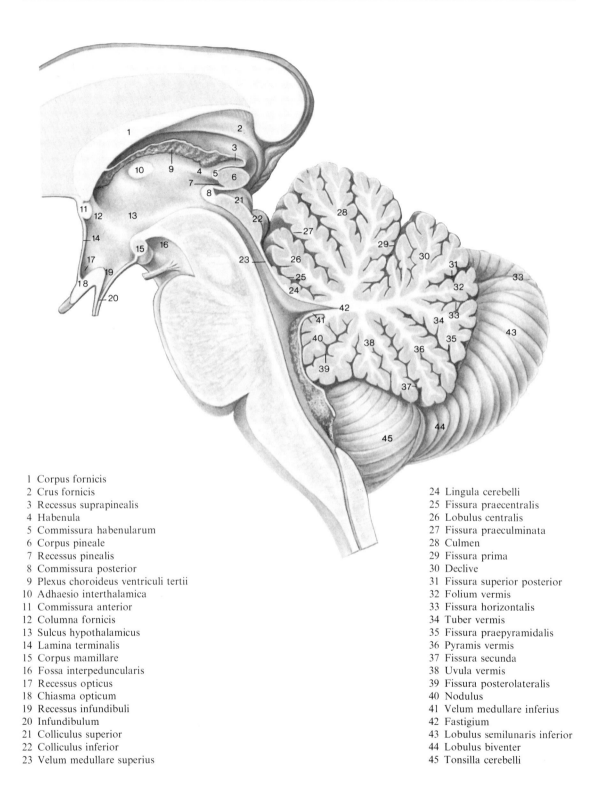

1 Corpus fornicis
2 Crus fornicis
3 Recessus suprapinealis
4 Habenula
5 Commissura habenularum
6 Corpus pineale
7 Recessus pinealis
8 Commissura posterior
9 Plexus choroideus ventriculi tertii
10 Adhaesio interthalamica
11 Commissura anterior
12 Columna fornicis
13 Sulcus hypothalamicus
14 Lamina terminalis
15 Corpus mamillare
16 Fossa interpeduncularis
17 Recessus opticus
18 Chiasma opticum
19 Recessus infundibuli
20 Infundibulum
21 Colliculus superior
22 Colliculus inferior
23 Velum medullare superius

24 Lingula cerebelli
25 Fissura praecentralis
26 Lobulus centralis
27 Fissura praeculminata
28 Culmen
29 Fissura prima
30 Declive
31 Fissura superior posterior
32 Folium vermis
33 Fissura horizontalis
34 Tuber vermis
35 Fissura praepyramidalis
36 Pyramis vermis
37 Fissura secunda
38 Uvula vermis
39 Fissura posterolateralis
40 Nodulus
41 Velum medullare inferius
42 Fastigium
43 Lobulus semilunaris inferior
44 Lobulus biventer
45 Tonsilla cerebelli

Fig. 13. Medial view of the bisected brain stem and cerebellum (3/2 ×)

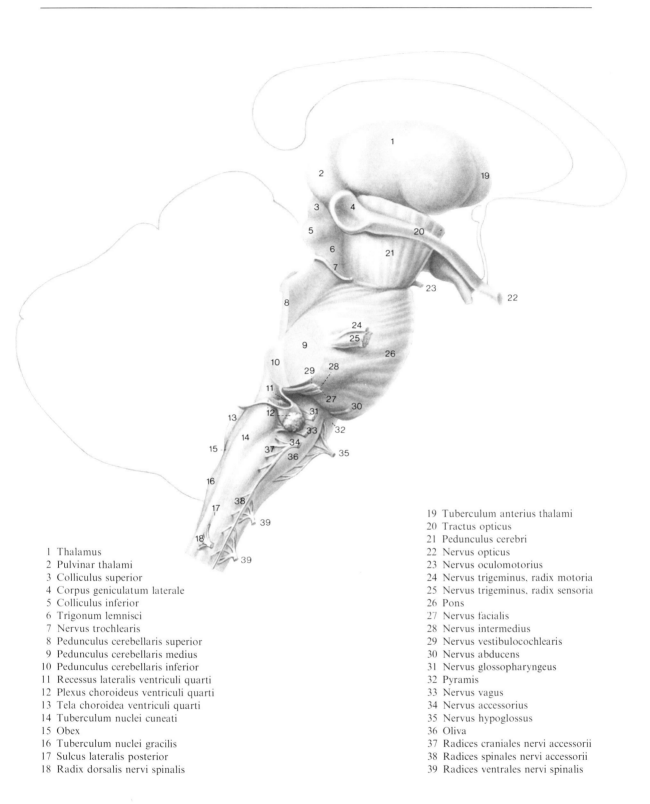

1 Thalamus
2 Pulvinar thalami
3 Colliculus superior
4 Corpus geniculatum laterale
5 Colliculus inferior
6 Trigonum lemnisci
7 Nervus trochlearis
8 Pedunculus cerebellaris superior
9 Pedunculus cerebellaris medius
10 Pedunculus cerebellaris inferior
11 Recessus lateralis ventriculi quarti
12 Plexus choroideus ventriculi quarti
13 Tela choroidea ventriculi quarti
14 Tuberculum nuclei cuneati
15 Obex
16 Tuberculum nuclei gracilis
17 Sulcus lateralis posterior
18 Radix dorsalis nervi spinalis

19 Tuberculum anterius thalami
20 Tractus opticus
21 Pedunculus cerebri
22 Nervus opticus
23 Nervus oculomotorius
24 Nervus trigeminus, radix motoria
25 Nervus trigeminus, radix sensoria
26 Pons
27 Nervus facialis
28 Nervus intermedius
29 Nervus vestibulocochlearis
30 Nervus abducens
31 Nervus glossopharyngeus
32 Pyramis
33 Nervus vagus
34 Nervus accessorius
35 Nervus hypoglossus
36 Oliva
37 Radices craniales nervi accessorii
38 Radices spinales nervi accessorii
39 Radices ventrales nervi spinalis

Fig. 14. Lateral view of the brain stem and the diencephalon after removal of the structures surrounding the thalamus (3/2 ×)

1 Ventriculus lateralis
2 Ventriculus tertius
3 Corpus pineale
4 Brachium colliculi superioris
5 Colliculus superior
6 Brachium colliculi inferioris
7 Colliculus inferior
8 Pedunculus cerebri

25 Taenia choroidea
26 Lamina affixa
27 Stria terminalis
28 Stria medullaris thalami
29 Taenia thalami
30 Trigonum habenulae
31 Pulvinar thalami
32 Corpus geniculatum mediale
33 Corpus geniculatum laterale

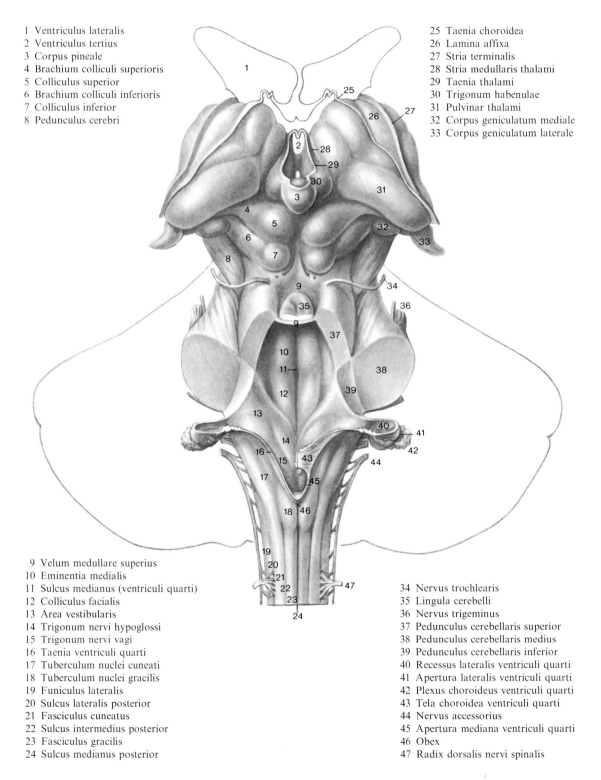

9 Velum medullare superius
10 Eminentia medialis
11 Sulcus medianus (ventriculi quarti)
12 Colliculus facialis
13 Area vestibularis
14 Trigonum nervi hypoglossi
15 Trigonum nervi vagi
16 Taenia ventriculi quarti
17 Tuberculum nuclei cuneati
18 Tuberculum nuclei gracilis
19 Funiculus lateralis
20 Sulcus lateralis posterior
21 Fasciculus cuneatus
22 Sulcus intermedius posterior
23 Fasciculus gracilis
24 Sulcus medianus posterior

34 Nervus trochlearis
35 Lingula cerebelli
36 Nervus trigeminus
37 Pedunculus cerebellaris superior
38 Pedunculus cerebellaris medius
39 Pedunculus cerebellaris inferior
40 Recessus lateralis ventriculi quarti
41 Apertura lateralis ventriculi quarti
42 Plexus choroideus ventriculi quarti
43 Tela choroidea ventriculi quarti
44 Nervus accessorius
45 Apertura mediana ventriculi quarti
46 Obex
47 Radix dorsalis nervi spinalis

Fig. 15. Dorsal view of the brain stem and the diencephalon after removal of the structures surrounding the thalamus. The contour of the cerebellum is indicated (3/2 ×)

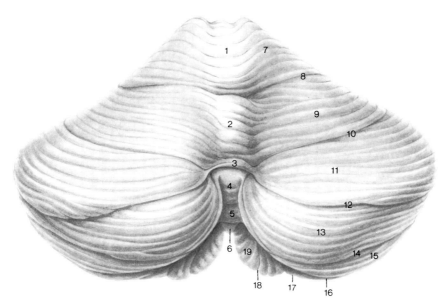

1 Culmen	7 Lobulus quadrangularis	13 Lobulus semilunaris inferior
2 Declive	8 Fissura prima	14 Fissura ansoparamediana
3 Folium vermis	9 Lobulus simplex	15 Lobulus gracilis
4 Tuber vermis	10 Fissura superior posterior	16 Fissura praebiventeris
5 Pyramis vermis	11 Lobulus semilunaris superior	17 Lobulus biventer
6 Uvula vermis	12 Fissura horizontalis	18 Fissura secunda
		19 Tonsilla cerebelli

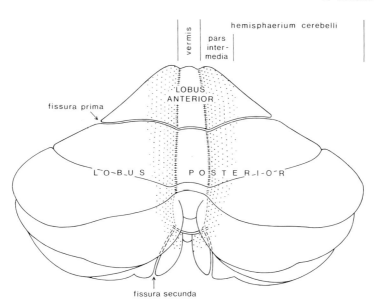

Fig. 16. Dorsal view of the cerebellum (6/5 ×; diagram: 1/1 ×)

1 Taenia choroidea
2 Lamina affixa
3 Taenia thalami
4 Tuberculum anterius thalami
5 Thalamus
6 Adhaesio interthalamica
7 Chiasma opticum
8 Nervus opticus
9 Tractus opticus
10 Corpus geniculatum laterale
11 Nervus oculomotorius
12 Nervus trochlearis

24 Ventriculus lateralis
25 Ventriculus tertius
26 Infundibulum
27 Corpus mamillare
28 Pedunculus cerebri
29 Substantia perforata posterior
30 Fossa interpeduncularis
31 Pons
32 Sulcus basilaris pontis

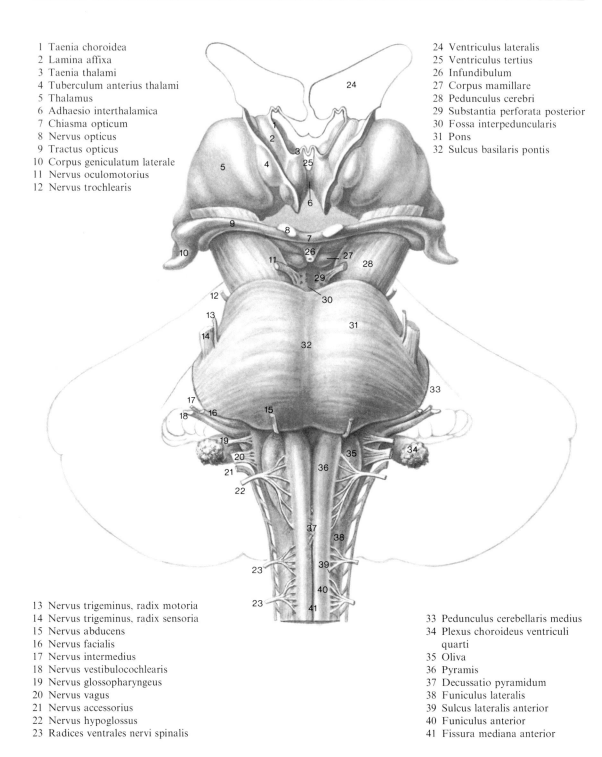

13 Nervus trigeminus, radix motoria
14 Nervus trigeminus, radix sensoria
15 Nervus abducens
16 Nervus facialis
17 Nervus intermedius
18 Nervus vestibulocochlearis
19 Nervus glossopharyngeus
20 Nervus vagus
21 Nervus accessorius
22 Nervus hypoglossus
23 Radices ventrales nervi spinalis

33 Pedunculus cerebellaris medius
34 Plexus choroideus ventriculi
   quarti
35 Oliva
36 Pyramis
37 Decussatio pyramidum
38 Funiculus lateralis
39 Sulcus lateralis anterior
40 Funiculus anterior
41 Fissura mediana anterior

Fig. 17. Ventral view of the brain stem and the diencephalon. The structures surrounding the thalamus have been removed (3/2 ×)

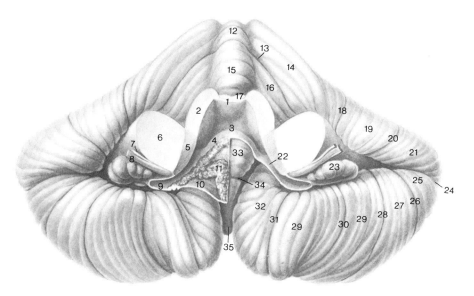

1 Velum medullare superius
2 Pedunculus cerebellaris superior
3 Fastigium
4 Velum medullare inferius
5 Pedunculus cerebellaris inferior
6 Pedunculus cerebellaris medius
7 Nervus intermedius
8 Nervus vestibulocochlearis
9 Recessus lateralis ventriculi quarti
10 Tela choroidea ventriculi quarti
11 Plexus choroideus ventriculi quarti

12 Culmen
13 Fissura praeculminata
14 Lobulus quadrangularis
15 Lobulus centralis
16 Ala lobuli centralis
17 Lingula cerebelli
18 Fissura prima
19 Lobulus simplex
20 Fissura superior posterior
21 Lobulus semilunaris superior
22 Pedunculus flocculi
23 Flocculus

24 Fissura horizontalis
25 Lobulus semilunaris inferior
26 Fissura ansoparamediana
27 Lobulus gracilis
28 Fissura praebiventeris
29 Lobulus biventer
30 Fissura intrabiventeris
31 Fissura secunda
32 Tonsilla cerebelli
33 Nodulus
34 Fissura posterolateralis
35 Uvula vermis

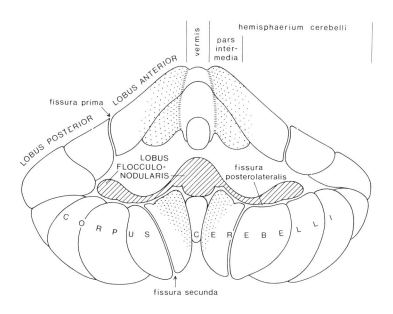

Fig. 18. Ventral view of the cerebellum (6/5 ×; diagram: 1/1 ×)

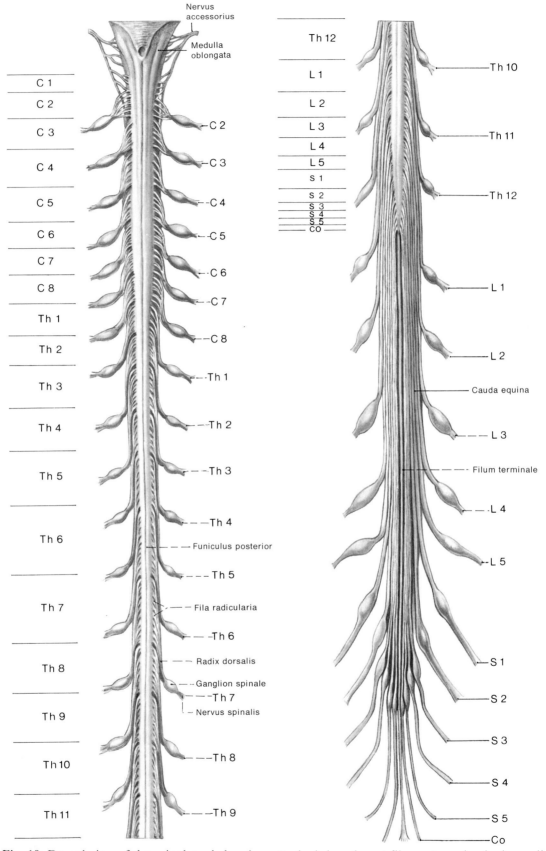

Fig. 19. Dorsal view of the spinal cord showing attached dorsal root filaments and spinal ganglia. The Cervical (*C*), Thoracic (*Th*), Lumbar (*L*), Sacral (*S*) and Coccygeal (*Co*) spinal nerves have been transected at their site of exit from the intervertebral foramina. The position of the spinal segments is indicated *left* to the cord (2/3 ×)

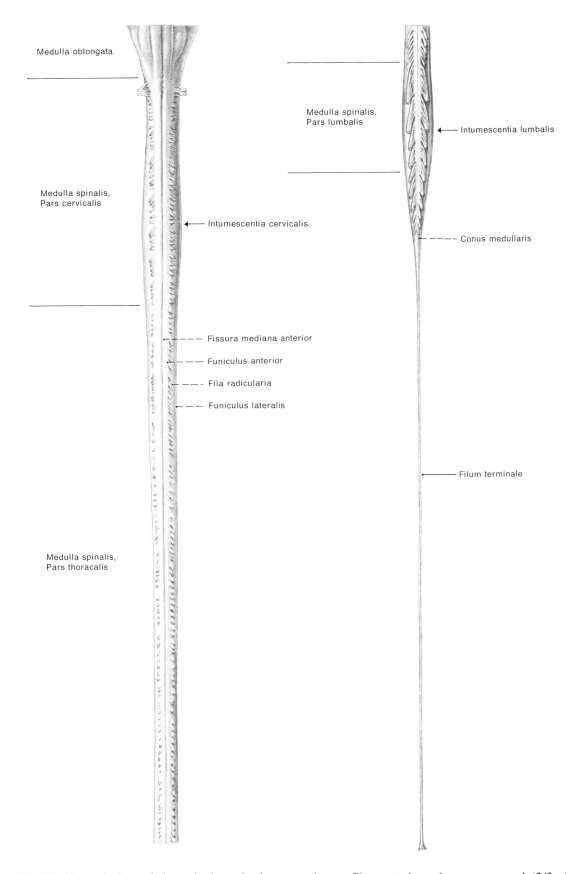

Medulla oblongata

Medulla spinalis,
Pars cervicalis

Medulla spinalis,
Pars thoracalis

Intumescentia cervicalis

Fissura mediana anterior

Funiculus anterior

Fila radicularia

Funiculus lateralis

Medulla spinalis,
Pars lumbalis

Intumescentia lumbalis

Conus medullaris

Filum terminale

Fig. 20. Ventral view of the spinal cord; the ventral root filaments have been transected (2/3 ×)

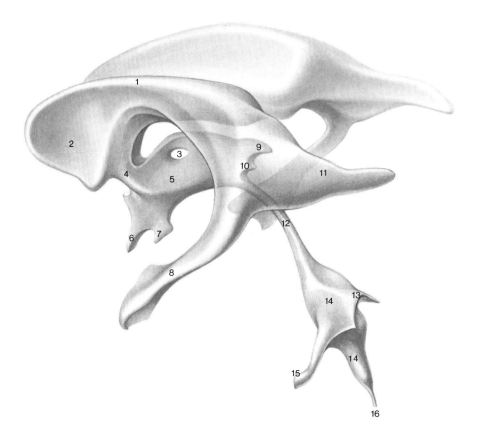

1 Ventriculus lateralis, pars centralis
2 Ventriculus lateralis, cornu anterius
3 Adhaesio interthalamica
4 Foramen interventriculare
5 Ventriculus tertius
6 Recessus opticus
7 Recessus infundibuli
8 Ventriculus lateralis, cornu inferius

9 Recessus suprapinealis
10 Recessus pinealis
11 Ventriculus lateralis, cornu posterius
12 Aqueductus cerebri
13 Fastigium
14 Ventriculus quartus
15 Recessus lateralis ventriculi quarti
16 Canalis centralis

Fig. 21. The ventricles of the brain; oblique view from behind and above (6/5 ×)

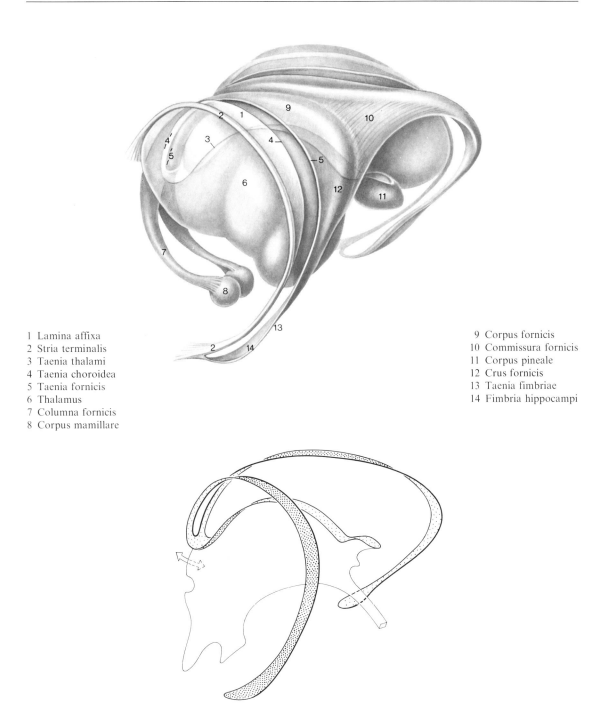

1 Lamina affixa
2 Stria terminalis
3 Taenia thalami
4 Taenia choroidea
5 Taenia fornicis
6 Thalamus
7 Columna fornicis
8 Corpus mamillare

9 Corpus fornicis
10 Commissura fornicis
11 Corpus pineale
12 Crus fornicis
13 Taenia fimbriae
14 Fimbria hippocampi

Fig. 22. Topography of diencephalic and telencephalic taeniae; oblique view from behind and above. In the complementary *diagram* the choroid walls of the lateral and third ventricles are shown. *Dense stippling*: ventricular surface; *light stippling*: meningeal surface; *double arrow*: interventricular foramen (2/1 ×; diagram: 5/3 ×)

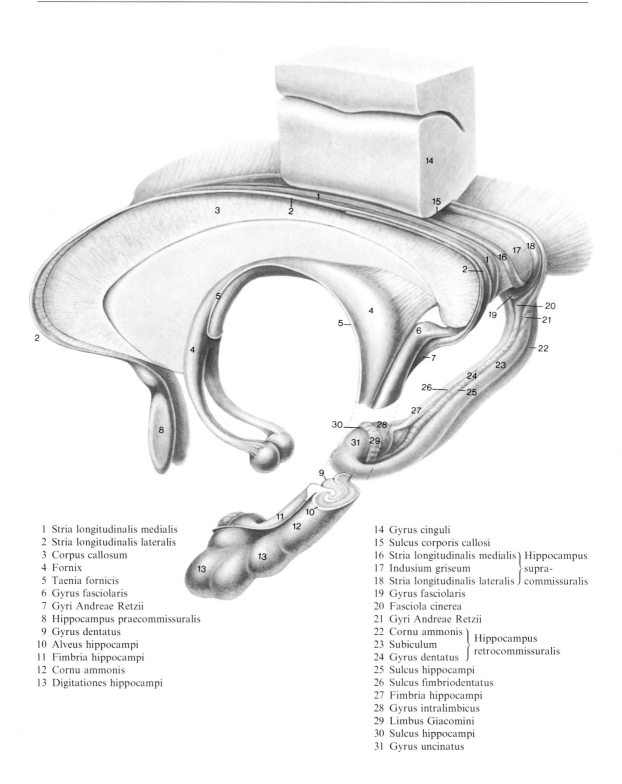

1 Stria longitudinalis medialis
2 Stria longitudinalis lateralis
3 Corpus callosum
4 Fornix
5 Taenia fornicis
6 Gyrus fasciolaris
7 Gyri Andreae Retzii
8 Hippocampus praecommissuralis
9 Gyrus dentatus
10 Alveus hippocampi
11 Fimbria hippocampi
12 Cornu ammonis
13 Digitationes hippocampi

14 Gyrus cinguli
15 Sulcus corporis callosi
16 Stria longitudinalis medialis ⎫ Hippocampus
17 Indusium griseum   ⎬ supra-
18 Stria longitudinalis lateralis ⎭ commissuralis
19 Gyrus fasciolaris
20 Fasciola cinerea
21 Gyri Andreae Retzii
22 Cornu ammonis ⎫ Hippocampus
23 Subiculum   ⎬ retrocommissuralis
24 Gyrus dentatus ⎭
25 Sulcus hippocampi
26 Sulcus fimbriodentatus
27 Fimbria hippocampi
28 Gyrus intralimbicus
29 Limbus Giacomini
30 Sulcus hippocampi
31 Gyrus uncinatus

Fig. 23. Dissection showing the hippocampus and some related structures in oblique view from behind and above (2/1 ×)

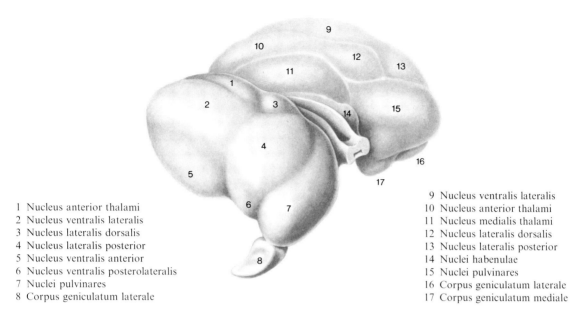

1 Nucleus anterior thalami
2 Nucleus ventralis lateralis
3 Nucleus lateralis dorsalis
4 Nucleus lateralis posterior
5 Nucleus ventralis anterior
6 Nucleus ventralis posterolateralis
7 Nuclei pulvinares
8 Corpus geniculatum laterale

9 Nucleus ventralis lateralis
10 Nucleus anterior thalami
11 Nucleus medialis thalami
12 Nucleus lateralis dorsalis
13 Nucleus lateralis posterior
14 Nuclei habenulae
15 Nuclei pulvinares
16 Corpus geniculatum laterale
17 Corpus geniculatum mediale

Fig. 24. A model of both thalami; oblique view from behind and above. The nucleus reticularis and the so-called midline nuclei have been omitted (2/1 ×)

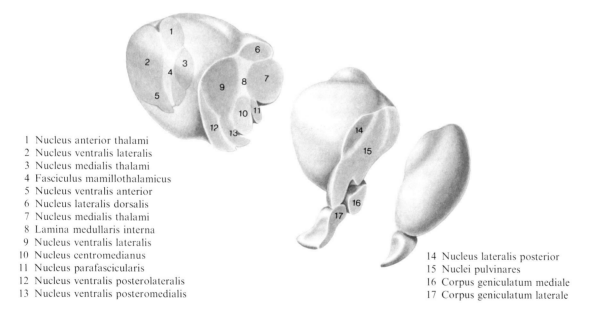

1 Nucleus anterior thalami
2 Nucleus ventralis lateralis
3 Nucleus medialis thalami
4 Fasciculus mamillothalamicus
5 Nucleus ventralis anterior
6 Nucleus lateralis dorsalis
7 Nucleus medialis thalami
8 Lamina medullaris interna
9 Nucleus ventralis lateralis
10 Nucleus centromedianus
11 Nucleus parafascicularis
12 Nucleus ventralis posterolateralis
13 Nucleus ventralis posteromedialis

14 Nucleus lateralis posterior
15 Nuclei pulvinares
16 Corpus geniculatum mediale
17 Corpus geniculatum laterale

Fig. 25. Left half of the same model as shown in Figure 24. The position of its major nuclei is indicated on three frontal sections (2/1 ×)

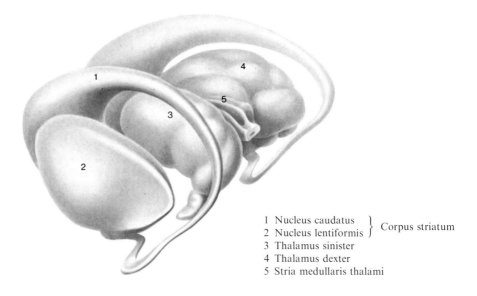

1 Nucleus caudatus   ⎫
2 Nucleus lentiformis   ⎬ Corpus striatum
3 Thalamus sinister   ⎭
4 Thalamus dexter
5 Stria medullaris thalami

Fig. 26. The corpus striatum and the thalamus of both sides in oblique view from behind and above (6/5 ×)

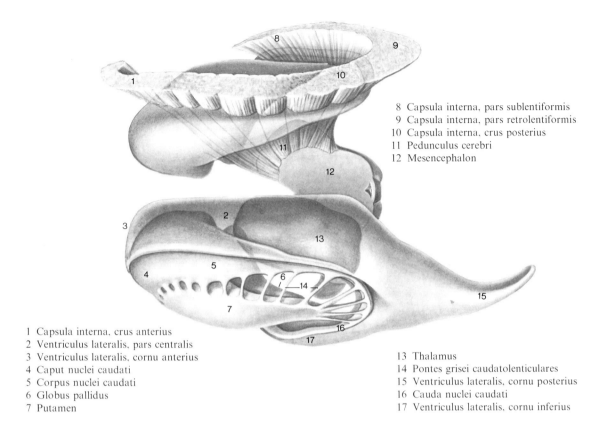

8 Capsula interna, pars sublentiformis
9 Capsula interna, pars retrolentiformis
10 Capsula interna, crus posterius
11 Pedunculus cerebri
12 Mesencephalon

1 Capsula interna, crus anterius
2 Ventriculus lateralis, pars centralis
3 Ventriculus lateralis, cornu anterius
4 Caput nuclei caudati
5 Corpus nuclei caudati
6 Globus pallidus
7 Putamen

13 Thalamus
14 Pontes grisei caudatolenticulares
15 Ventriculus lateralis, cornu posterius
16 Cauda nuclei caudati
17 Ventriculus lateralis, cornu inferius

Fig. 27. The corpus striatum of both sides, viewed from above. The thalamus and the extent of the lateral ventricle can be seen on the *left side*. The internal capsule and its convergence upon the pedunculus cerebri are indicated on the *right side* (6/5 ×)

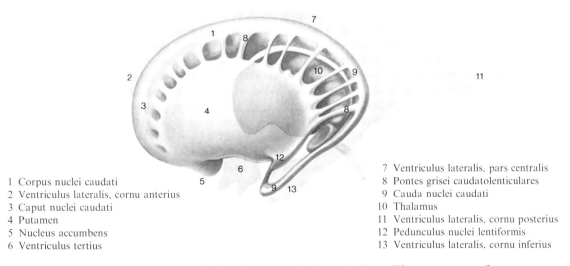

1 Corpus nuclei caudati
2 Ventriculus lateralis, cornu anterius
3 Caput nuclei caudati
4 Putamen
5 Nucleus accumbens
6 Ventriculus tertius

7 Ventriculus lateralis, pars centralis
8 Pontes grisei caudatolenticulares
9 Cauda nuclei caudati
10 Thalamus
11 Ventriculus lateralis, cornu posterius
12 Pedunculus nuclei lentiformis
13 Ventriculus lateralis, cornu inferius

Fig. 28. The corpus striatum and the thalamus in lateral view. The contours of some parts of the ventricular system are indicated (6/5 ×)

Part II Brain Slices

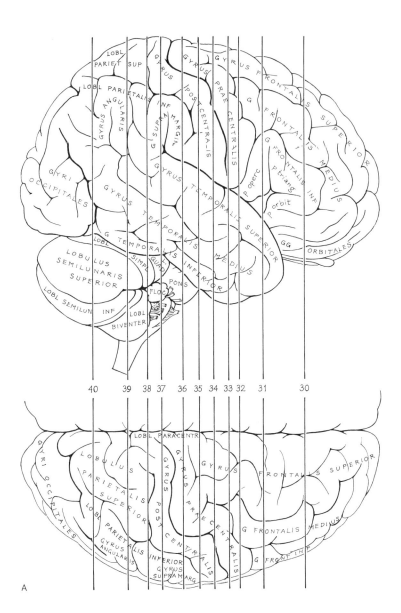

LOBL PARIET SUP
LOBL PARIETALIS INF
GYRUS ANGULARIS
GYRI OCCIPITALES
GYRUS TEMPORALIS
G TEMPORALIS
LOBULUS SEMILUNARIS SUPERIOR
LOBL SEMILUN INF
LOBL BIVENTER
LOBL SIMPL
QUADR
FLOC
PONS
GYRUS SUPRA MARGIN
G TEMPORALIS INFERIOR
GYRUS POST CENTRALIS
GYRUS TEMPORALIS SUPERIOR
GYRUS TEMPORALIS MEDIUS
GYRUS PRAE CENTRALIS
GYRUS FRONTALIS SUPERIOR
G FRONTALIS MEDIUS
G FRONTALIS INF
P operc
P triang
P orbit
GG ORBITALES

40 39 38 37 36 35 34 33 32 31   30

LOBL PARACENTR
LOBULUS PARIETALIS SUPERIOR
GYRI OCCIPITALES
LOBL PARIETALIS INFERIOR
GYRUS ANGULARIS
GYRUS SUPRAMARG
GYRUS POST CENTRALIS
GYRUS PRAE CENTRALIS
GYRUS FRONTALIS SUPERIOR
G FRONTALIS MEDIUS
G FRONT INF

A

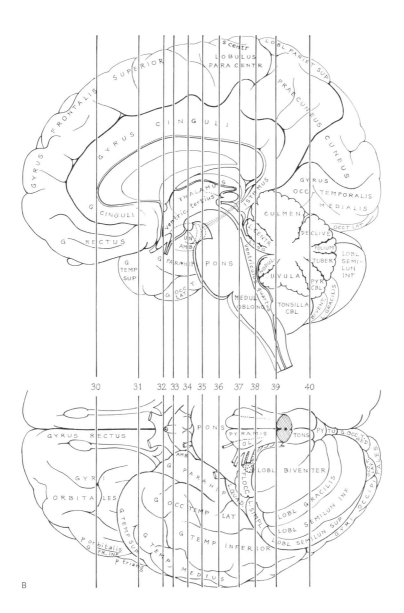

Fig. 29A and B. Key diagrams showing the level and plane of the coronal sections in Figures 30–40 (2/3 ×)

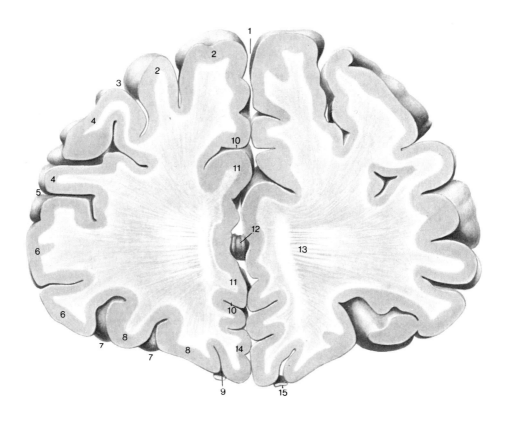

1 Fissura longitudinalis cerebri
2 Gyrus frontalis superior
3 Sulcus frontalis superior
4 Gyrus frontalis medius
5 Sulcus frontalis inferior
6 Gyrus frontalis inferior
7 Sulci orbitales
8 Gyri orbitales
9 Sulcus olfactorius

10 Sulcus cinguli
11 Gyrus cinguli
12 Genu corporis callosi
13 Radiatio corporis callosi
14 Gyrus rectus
15 Tractus olfactorius

Fig. 30. Section through the anterior part of the cerebral hemispheres (6/5 ×)

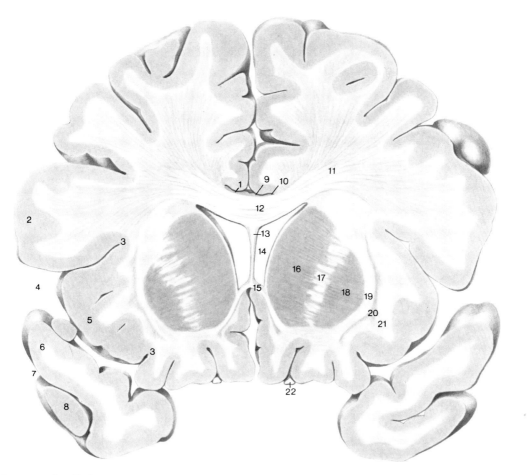

1 Sulcus corporis callosi
2 Gyrus frontalis inferior
3 Sulcus circularis insulae
4 Sulcus lateralis
5 Gyri breves insulae
6 Gyrus temporalis superior
7 Sulcus temporalis superior
8 Gyrus temporalis medius

9 Stria longitudinalis medialis
10 Stria longitudinalis lateralis
11 Radiatio corporis callosi
12 Truncus corporis callosi
13 Septum pellucidum
14 Ventriculus lateralis, cornu anterius
15 Rostrum corporis callosi
16 Caput nuclei caudati
17 Capsula interna, crus anterius
18 Putamen
19 Capsula externa
20 Claustrum
21 Capsula extrema
22 Tractus olfactorius

Fig. 31. Section through the head of the caudate nucleus and the putamen (6/5 ×)

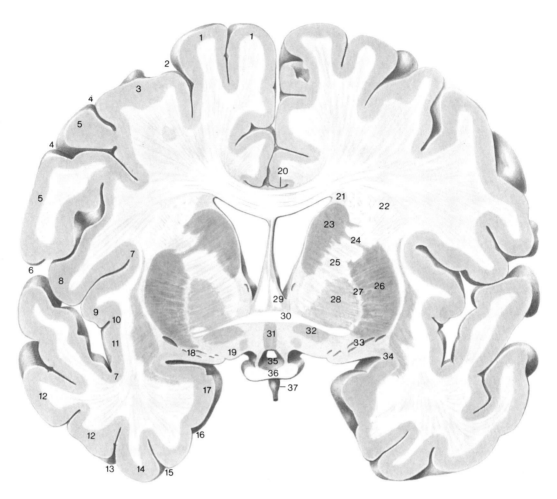

1 Gyrus frontalis superior
2 Sulcus frontalis superior
3 Gyrus frontalis medius
4 Sulcus praecentralis
5 Gyrus praecentralis
6 Sulcus lateralis, ramus posterior
7 Sulcus circularis insulae
8 Gyrus frontalis inferior, pars opercularis
9 Gyri breves insulae
10 Sulcus centralis insulae
11 Gyrus longus insulae
12 Gyrus temporalis medius
13 Sulcus temporalis inferior
14 Gyrus occipitotemporalis lateralis
15 Sulcus collateralis
16 Sulcus rhinalis
17 Gyrus parahippocampalis
18 Substantia perforata anterior
19 Gyrus diagonalis

20 Indusium griseum
21 Stratum subependymale
22 Corona radiata
23 Caput nuclei caudati
24 Pontes grisei caudatolenticulares
25 Capsula interna, crus anterius
26 Putamen
27 Lamina medullaris lateralis
28 Globus pallidus
29 Columna fornicis
30 Commissura anterior
31 Lamina terminalis
32 Substantia innominata
33 Arteria cerebri media, rami striati
34 Stria olfactoria lateralis
35 Recessus opticus
36 Chiasma opticum
37 Infundibulum

Fig. 32. Section through the anterior commissure and the optic chiasm (6/5 ×)

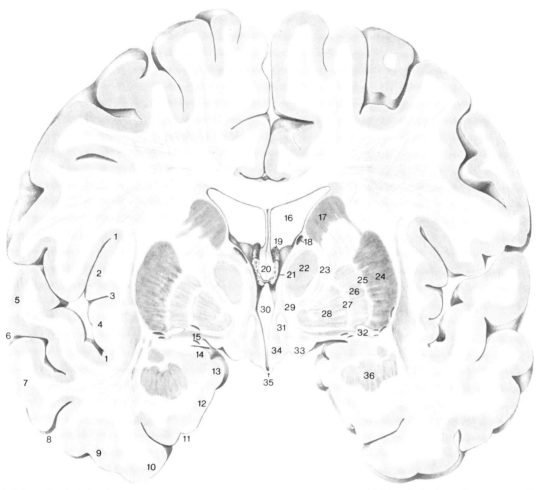

1 Sulcus circularis insulae
2 Gyri breves insulae
3 Sulcus centralis insulae
4 Gyrus longus insulae
5 Gyrus temporalis superior
6 Sulcus temporalis superior
7 Gyrus temporalis medius
8 Sulcus temporalis inferior
9 Gyrus temporalis inferior
10 Gyrus occipitotemporalis lateralis
11 Sulcus rhinalis
12 Gyrus parahippocampalis
13 Gyrus ambiens
14 Gyrus semilunaris
15 Arteria cerebri media, rami striati

16 Ventriculus lateralis, pars centralis
17 Corpus nuclei caudati
18 Vena thalamostriata
19 Plexus choroideus ventriculi lateralis
20 Corpus fornicis
21 Foramen interventriculare
22 Nucleus anterior thalami
23 Capsula interna, genu
24 Putamen
25 Lamina medullaris lateralis
26 Globus pallidus, pars lateralis
27 Lamina medullaris medialis
28 Globus pallidus, pars medialis
29 Pedunculus thalami inferior
30 Ventriculus tertius
31 Columna fornicis
32 Commissura anterior
33 Tractus opticus
34 Hypothalamus
35 Infundibulum
36 Corpus amygdaloideum

Fig. 33. Section through the interventricular foramen, the infundibulum and the amygdaloid body (6/5 ×)

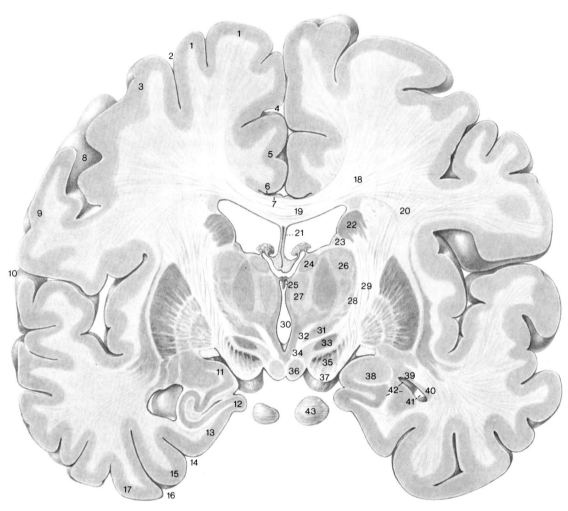

1 Gyrus frontalis superior	18 Radiatio corporis callosi	26 Nucleus ventralis lateralis
2 Sulcus praecentralis	19 Truncus corporis callosi	27 Nucleus medialis thalami
3 Gyrus praecentralis	20 Corona radiata	28 Nucleus reticularis thalami
4 Sulcus cinguli	21 Septum pellucidum	29 Capsula interna, crus posterius
5 Gyrus cinguli	22 Corpus nuclei caudati	30 Ventriculus tertius
6 Sulcus corporis callosi	23 Stria terminalis	31 Zona incerta
7 Indusium griseum	24 Nucleus anterior	32 Tractus mamillothalamicus
8 Sulcus centralis	thalami	33 Nucleus subthalamicus
9 Gyrus postcentralis	25 Plexus choroideus	34 Fasciculus mamillaris princeps
10 Sulcus lateralis, ramus posterior	ventriculi tertii	35 Substantia nigra
11 Gyrus uncinatus		36 Corpus mamillare
12 Gyrus ambiens		37 Pedunculus cerebri
13 Gyrus parahippocampalis		38 Corpus amygdaloideum
14 Sulcus collateralis		39 Stria terminalis
15 Gyrus occipitotemporalis lateralis		40 Cauda nuclei caudati
16 Sulcus occipitotemporalis		41 Ventriculus lateralis, cornu inferius
17 Gyrus temporalis inferior		42 Pes hippocampi
		43 Pons

Fig. 34. Section through the anterior end of the hippocampus, the mamillary body and the mamillothalamic tract (6/5 ×)

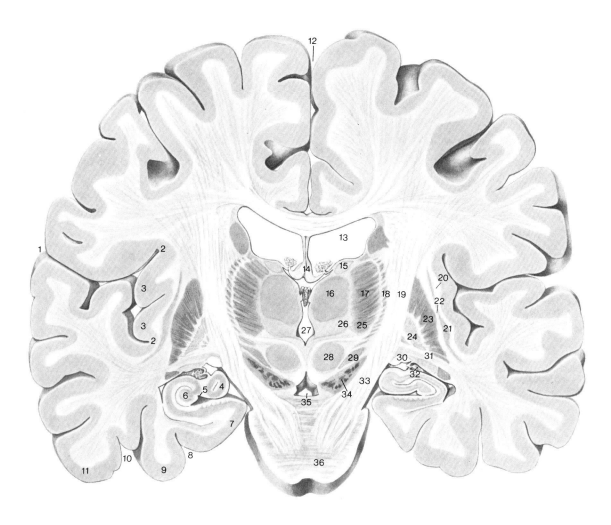

1 Sulcus lateralis, ramus posterior
2 Sulcus circularis insulae
3 Gyrus longus insulae
4 Gyrus intralimbicus
5 Sulcus hippocampi
6 Gyrus dentatus
7 Gyrus parahippocampalis
8 Sulcus collateralis
9 Gyrus occipitotemporalis lateralis
10 Sulcus occipitotemporalis
11 Gyrus temporalis inferior

12 Fissura longitudinalis cerebri
13 Ventriculus lateralis,
    pars centralis
14 Corpus fornicis
15 Nucleus lateralis dorsalis
16 Nucleus medialis thalami
17 Nucleus ventralis lateralis

18 Nucleus reticularis thalami
19 Capsula interna, crus posterius
20 Capsula extrema
21 Claustrum
22 Capsula externa
23 Putamen
24 Globus pallidus
25 Nucleus ventralis posterolateralis
26 Nucleus centromedianus
27 Ventriculus tertius
28 Nucleus ruber
29 Nucleus subthalamicus
30 Tractus opticus
31 Capsula interna, pars sublentiformis
32 Plexus choroideus ventriculi lateralis
33 Pedunculus cerebri
34 Substantia nigra
35 Fossa interpeduncularis
36 Pons

Fig. 35. Section through the thalamus, the cerebral peduncle and the pons (6/5 ×)

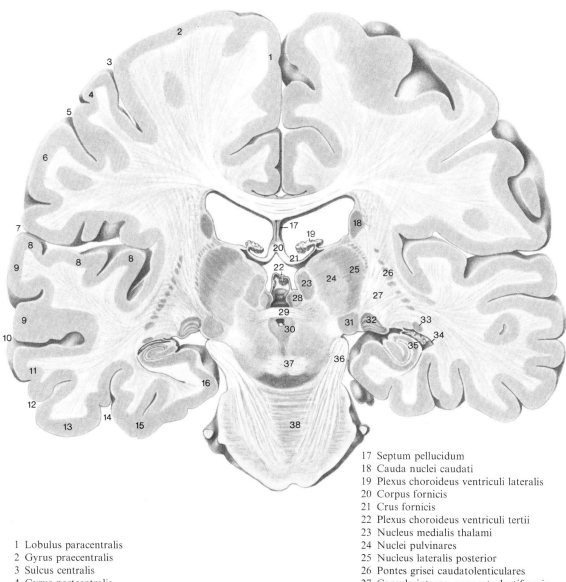

17 Septum pellucidum
18 Cauda nuclei caudati
19 Plexus choroideus ventriculi lateralis
20 Corpus fornicis
21 Crus fornicis
22 Plexus choroideus ventriculi tertii
23 Nucleus medialis thalami
24 Nuclei pulvinares
25 Nucleus lateralis posterior
26 Pontes grisei caudatolenticulares
27 Capsula interna, pars retrolentiformis
28 Nuclei habenulae
29 Commissura posterior
30 Aqueductus cerebri
31 Corpus geniculatum mediale
32 Corpus geniculatum laterale
33 Cauda nuclei caudati
34 Ventriculus lateralis, cornu inferius
35 Hippocampus
36 Pedunculus cerebri
37 Decussatio pedunculorum cerebellarium
   superiorum
38 Pons

 1 Lobulus paracentralis
 2 Gyrus praecentralis
 3 Sulcus centralis
 4 Gyrus postcentralis
 5 Sulcus postcentralis
 6 Lobulus parietalis inferior
 7 Sulcus lateralis, ramus posterior
 8 Gyri temporales transversi (Heschl)
 9 Gyrus temporalis superior
10 Sulcus temporalis superior
11 Gyrus temporalis medius
12 Sulcus temporalis inferior
13 Gyrus temporalis inferior
14 Sulcus occipitotemporalis
15 Gyrus occipitotemporalis lateralis
16 Gyrus parahippocampalis

Fig. 36. Section through the posterior part of the thalamus (6/5 ×)

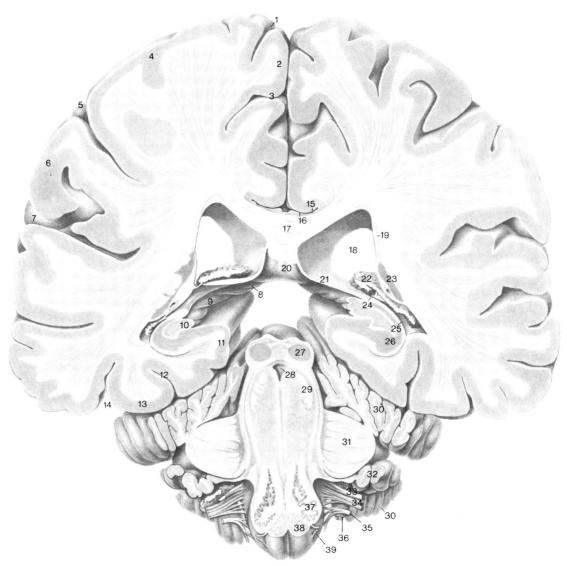

1 Sulcus centralis
2 Lobulus paracentralis
3 Sulcus cinguli, pars marginalis
4 Gyrus postcentralis
5 Sulcus postcentralis
6 Lobulus parietalis inferior
7 Sulcus lateralis, ramus posterior
8 Gyrus fasciolaris
9 Fasciola cinerea
10 Gyrus dentatus
11 Gyrus parahippocampalis
12 Sulcus collateralis
13 Gyrus occipitotemporalis lateralis
14 Sulcus occipitotemporalis

15 Sulcus corporis callosi
16 Indusium griseum
17 Truncus corporis callosi
18 Ventriculus lateralis
19 Stratum subependymale
20 Splenium corporis callosi
21 Crus fornicis
22 Plexus choroideus ventriculi
   lateralis
23 Cauda nuclei caudati
24 Fimbria hippocampi
25 Alveus hippocampi
26 Hippocampus

27 Colliculus inferior
28 Aqueductus cerebri
29 Pedunculus cerebellaris superior
30 Hemisphaerium cerebelli
31 Pedunculus cerebellaris medius
32 Flocculus
33 Nervus glossopharyngeus
34 Nervus vagus
35 Nervus accessorius
36 Plexus choroideus ventriculi quarti
37 Oliva
38 Pyramis
39 Nervus hypoglossus

Fig. 37. Section through the inferior colliculus and the inferior olive. The thickness of this slice is three times the standard of 2 mm (6/5 ×)

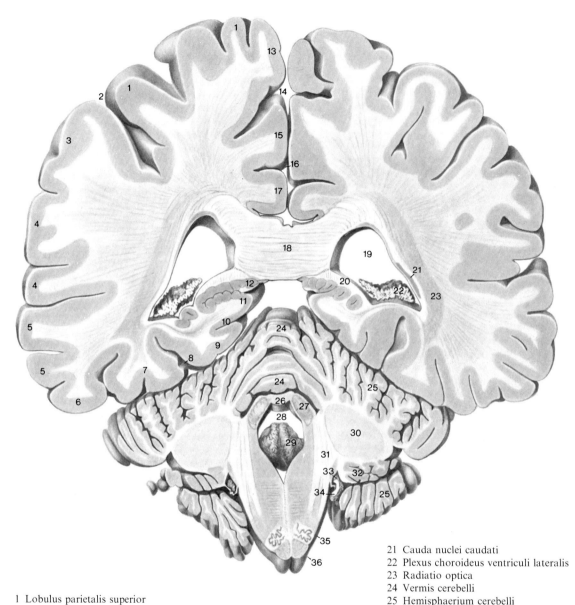

1 Lobulus parietalis superior
2 Sulcus intraparietalis
3 Lobulus parietalis inferior
4 Gyrus temporalis superior
5 Gyrus temporalis medius
6 Gyrus temporalis inferior
7 Gyrus occipitotemporalis lateralis
8 Sulcus collateralis
9 Gyrus occipitotemporalis medialis
10 Sulcus calcarinus
11 Isthmus gyri cinguli
12 Gyrus fasciolaris

13 Lobulus paracentralis
14 Sulcus cinguli,
   pars marginalis
15 Praecuneus
16 Sulcus subparietalis
17 Gyrus cinguli
18 Splenium corporis callosi
19 Ventriculus lateralis
20 Fimbria hippocampi

21 Cauda nuclei caudati
22 Plexus choroideus ventriculi lateralis
23 Radiatio optica
24 Vermis cerebelli
25 Hemisphaerium cerebelli
26 Velum medullare superius
27 Pedunculus cerebellaris superior
28 Ventriculus quartus
29 Plexus choroideus ventriculi quarti
30 Pedunculus cerebellaris medius
31 Pedunculus cerebellaris inferior
32 Flocculus
33 Recessus lateralis ventriculi quarti
34 Plexus choroideus ventriculi quarti
35 Oliva
36 Pyramis

Fig. 38. Section through the splenium of the corpus callosum and the fourth ventricle (6/5 ×)

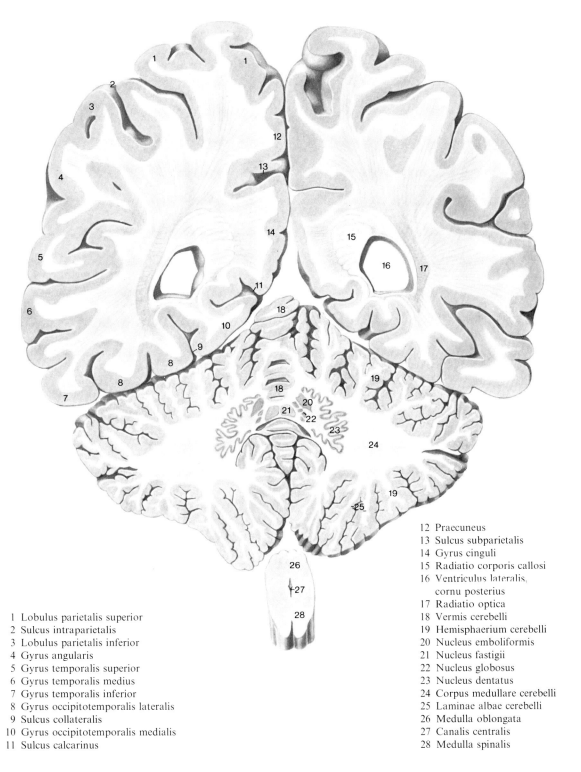

1 Lobulus parietalis superior
2 Sulcus intraparietalis
3 Lobulus parietalis inferior
4 Gyrus angularis
5 Gyrus temporalis superior
6 Gyrus temporalis medius
7 Gyrus temporalis inferior
8 Gyrus occipitotemporalis lateralis
9 Sulcus collateralis
10 Gyrus occipitotemporalis medialis
11 Sulcus calcarinus

12 Praecuneus
13 Sulcus subparietalis
14 Gyrus cinguli
15 Radiatio corporis callosi
16 Ventriculus lateralis,
   cornu posterius
17 Radiatio optica
18 Vermis cerebelli
19 Hemisphaerium cerebelli
20 Nucleus emboliformis
21 Nucleus fastigii
22 Nucleus globosus
23 Nucleus dentatus
24 Corpus medullare cerebelli
25 Laminae albae cerebelli
26 Medulla oblongata
27 Canalis centralis
28 Medulla spinalis

Fig. 39. Section through the posterior horns of the lateral ventricles and the central cerebellar nuclei (6/5 ×)

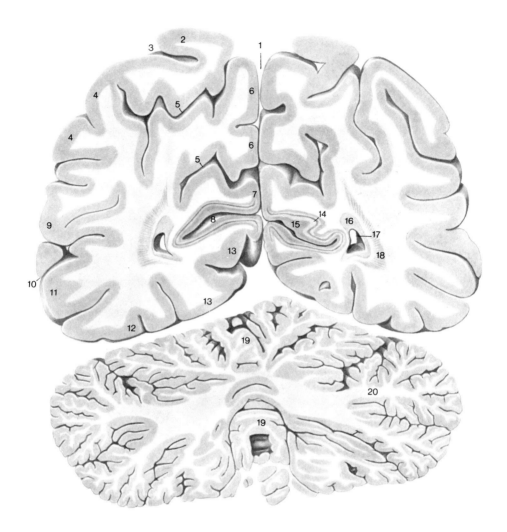

1 Fissura longitudinalis cerebri
2 Lobulus parietalis superior
3 Sulcus intraparietalis
4 Lobulus parietalis inferior
5 Sulcus parieto-occipitalis
6 Praecuneus
7 Cuneus
8 Sulcus calcarinus
9 Gyrus temporalis medius
10 Sulcus occipitalis anterior
11 Gyri occipitales
12 Gyrus occipitotemporalis lateralis
13 Gyrus occipitotemporalis medialis

14 Stria Gennari
15 Area striata
16 Radiatio corporis callosi
17 Ventriculus lateralis, cornu posterius
18 Radiatio optica
19 Vermis cerebelli
20 Hemisphaerium cerebelli

Fig. 40. Section through the deepest part of the calcarine sulcus (6/5 ×)

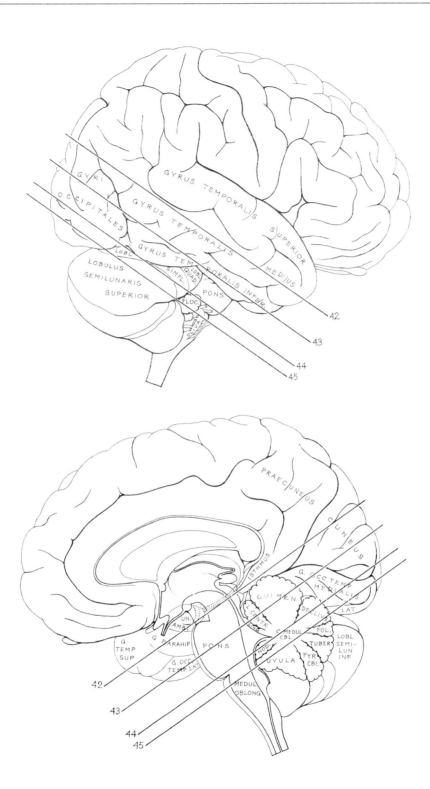

Fig. 41. Key diagrams showing the level and plane of the sections perpendicular to the axis of the brain stem in Figures 42–45 (2/3 ×)

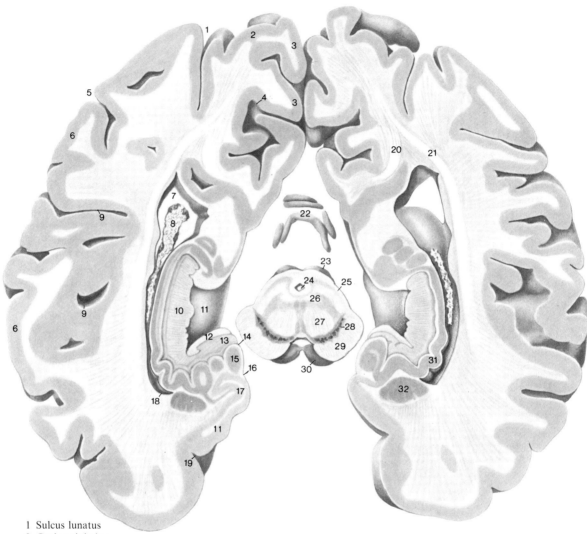

1 Sulcus lunatus
2 Gyri occipitales
3 Cuneus
4 Sulcus parieto-occipitalis
5 Sulcus occipitalis anterior
6 Gyrus temporalis medius
7 Ventriculus lateralis, cornu posterius
8 Plexus choroideus ventriculi lateralis
9 Sulcus temporalis superior
10 Gyrus dentatus
11 Gyrus parahippocampalis
12 Gyrus intralimbicus
13 Limbus Giacomini
14 Sulcus hippocampi
15 Gyrus uncinatus
16 Incisura unci
17 Gyrus ambiens
18 Ventriculus lateralis, cornu inferius
19 Sulcus rhinalis

20 Radiatio corporis callosi
21 Radiatio optica
22 Culmen
23 Colliculus inferior
24 Aqueductus cerebri
25 Brachium colliculi inferioris
26 Tegmentum mesencephali
27 Pedunculus cerebellaris superior
28 Substantia nigra
29 Pedunculus cerebri
30 Pons
31 Cornu ammonis
32 Corpus amygdaloideum

Fig. 42. Section through the middle of the midbrain (6/5 ×)

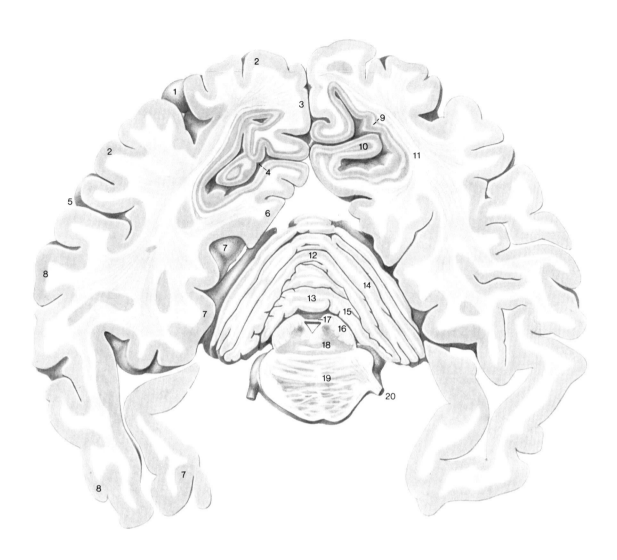

1 Sulcus lunatus
2 Gyri occipitales
3 Cuneus
4 Sulcus calcarinus
5 Sulcus occipitalis anterior
6 Gyrus occipitotemporalis medialis
7 Gyrus occipitotemporalis lateralis
8 Gyrus temporalis inferior

9 Stria Gennari
10 Area striata
11 Radiatio optica
12 Culmen
13 Lobulus centralis
14 Lobulus quadrangularis
15 Ala lobuli centralis
16 Pedunculus cerebellaris superior
17 Velum medullare superius
18 Tegmentum pontis
19 Pons
20 Nervus trigeminus

Fig. 43. Section through the pons at the level of the entrance of the trigeminal nerve (6/5×)

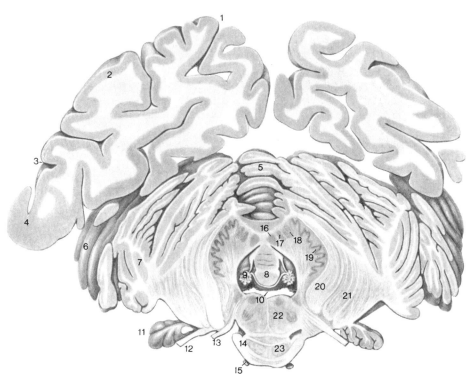

1 Sulcus calcarinus
2 Gyri occipitales
3 Sulcus occipitalis anterior
4 Gyrus temporalis inferior
5 Declive
6 Lobulus semilunaris superior
7 Lobulus simplex
8 Nodulus
9 Plexus choroideus ventriculi quarti
10 Ventriculus quartus
11 Flocculus
12 Nervus vestibulocochlearis
13 Nervus facialis
14 Pons
15 Nervus abducens

16 Nucleus fastigii
17 Nucleus globosus
18 Nucleus emboliformis
19 Nucleus dentatus
20 Pedunculus cerebellaris inferior
21 Pedunculus cerebellaris medius
22 Tegmentum pontis
23 Tractus corticospinalis

Fig. 44. Section through the transitional area of pons and medulla oblongata (6/5 ×)

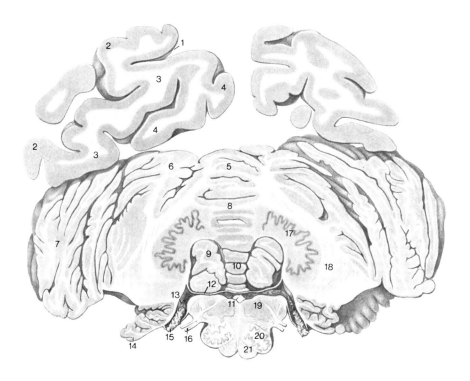

1 Sulcus calcarinus
2 Gyri occipitales
3 Gyrus occipitotemporalis lateralis
4 Gyrus occipitotemporalis medialis
5 Declive
6 Lobulus simplex
7 Lobulus semilunaris superior
8 Pyramis vermis
9 Tonsilla cerebelli
10 Uvula vermis
11 Ventriculus quartus
12 Tela choroidea ventriculi quarti
13 Recessus lateralis ventriculi quarti
14 Flocculus
15 Plexus choroideus ventriculi quarti
16 Nervus glossopharyngeus

17 Nucleus dentatus
18 Pedunculus cerebellaris medius
19 Tegmentum myelencephali
20 Nucleus olivaris inferior
21 Tractus corticospinalis

Fig. 45. Section through the medulla oblongata (6/5 ×)

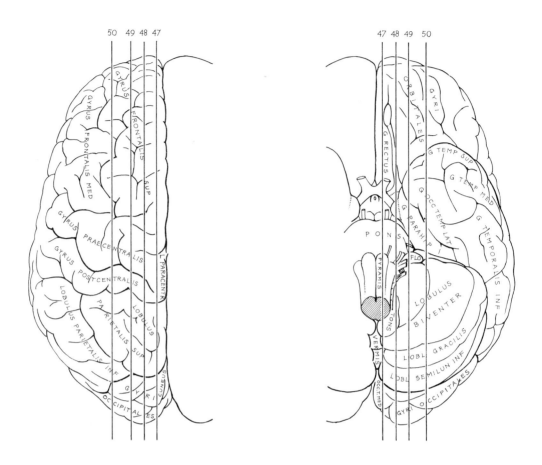

Fig. 46. Key diagrams showing the level and plane of the sagittal sections in Figures 47–50 (2/3 ×)

Fig. 47. Section through the mamillary body, the red nucleus and the fornix (6/5 ×)

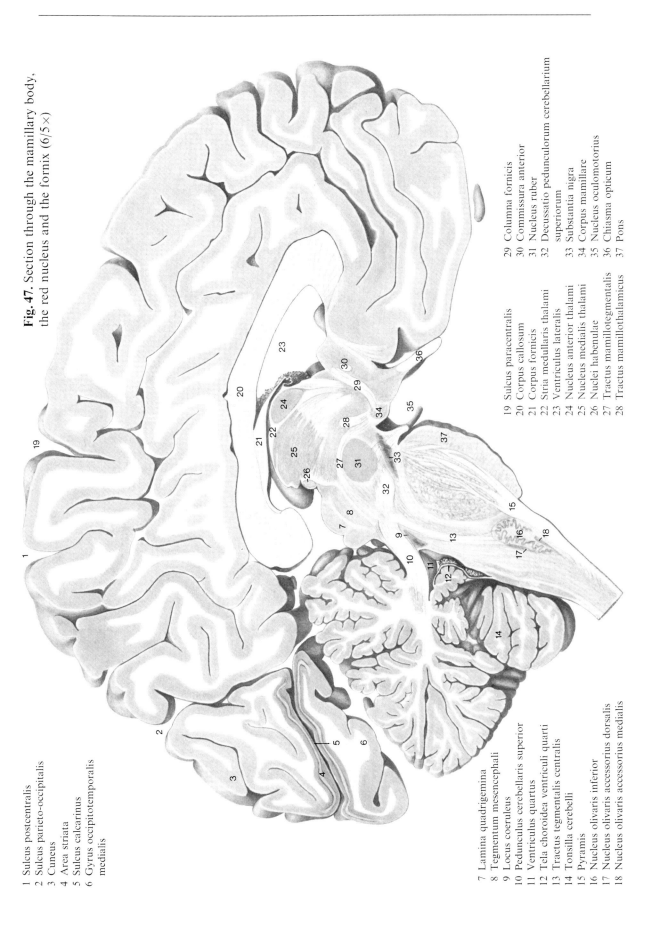

1 Sulcus postcentralis
2 Sulcus parieto-occipitalis
3 Cuneus
4 Area striata
5 Sulcus calcarinus
6 Gyrus occipitotemporalis medialis

7 Lamina quadrigemina
8 Tegmentum mesencephali
9 Locus coeruleus
10 Pedunculus cerebellaris superior
11 Ventriculus quartus
12 Tela choroidea ventriculi quarti
13 Tractus tegmentalis centralis
14 Tonsilla cerebelli
15 Pyramis
16 Nucleus olivaris inferior
17 Nucleus olivaris accessorius dorsalis
18 Nucleus olivaris accessorius medialis

19 Sulcus paracentralis
20 Corpus callosum
21 Corpus fornicis
22 Stria medullaris thalami
23 Ventriculus lateralis
24 Nucleus anterior thalami
25 Nucleus medialis thalami
26 Nuclei habenulae
27 Tractus mamillotegmentalis
28 Tractus mamillothalamicus

29 Columna fornicis
30 Commissura anterior
31 Nucleus ruber
32 Decussatio pedunculorum cerebellarium
   superiorum
33 Substantia nigra
34 Corpus mamillare
35 Nucleus oculomotorius
36 Chiasma opticum
37 Pons

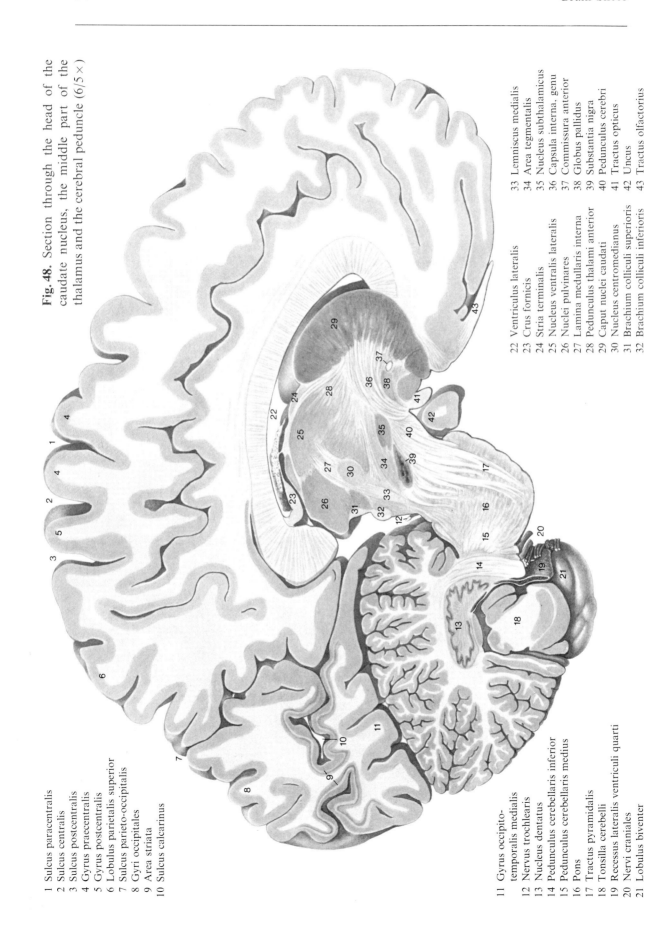

Fig. 48. Section through the head of the caudate nucleus, the middle part of the thalamus and the cerebral peduncle (6/5 ×)

1 Sulcus paracentralis
2 Sulcus centralis
3 Sulcus postcentralis
4 Gyrus praecentralis
5 Gyrus postcentralis
6 Lobulus parietalis superior
7 Sulcus parieto-occipitalis
8 Gyri occipitales
9 Area striata
10 Sulcus calcarinus

11 Gyrus occipito-
   temporalis medialis
12 Nervus trochlearis
13 Nucleus dentatus
14 Pedunculus cerebellaris inferior
15 Pedunculus cerebellaris medius
16 Pons
17 Tractus pyramidalis
18 Tonsilla cerebelli
19 Recessus lateralis ventriculi quarti
20 Nervi craniales
21 Lobulus biventer

22 Ventriculus lateralis
23 Crus fornicis
24 Stria terminalis
25 Nucleus ventralis lateralis
26 Nuclei pulvinares
27 Lamina medullaris interna
28 Pedunculus thalami anterior
29 Caput nuclei caudati
30 Nucleus centromedianus
31 Brachium colliculi superioris
32 Brachium colliculi inferioris

33 Lemniscus medialis
34 Area tegmentalis
35 Nucleus subthalamicus
36 Capsula interna, genu
37 Commissura anterior
38 Globus pallidus
39 Substantia nigra
40 Pedunculus cerebri
41 Tractus opticus
42 Uncus
43 Tractus olfactorius

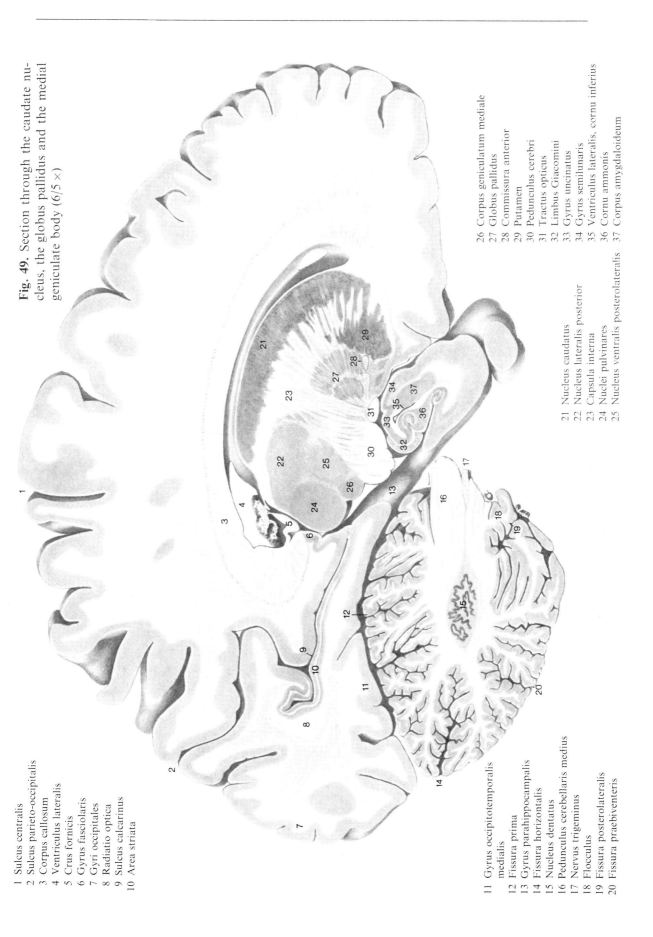

Fig. 49. Section through the caudate nucleus, the globus pallidus and the medial geniculate body (6/5 ×)

1 Sulcus centralis
2 Sulcus parieto-occipitalis
3 Corpus callosum
4 Ventriculus lateralis
5 Crus fornicis
6 Gyrus fasciolaris
7 Gyri occipitales
8 Radiatio optica
9 Sulcus calcarinus
10 Area striata

11 Gyrus occipitotemporalis medialis
12 Fissura prima
13 Gyrus parahippocampalis
14 Fissura horizontalis
15 Nucleus dentatus
16 Pedunculus cerebellaris medius
17 Nervus trigeminus
18 Flocculus
19 Fissura posterolateralis
20 Fissura praebiventeris

21 Nucleus caudatus
22 Nucleus lateralis posterior
23 Capsula interna
24 Nuclei pulvinares
25 Nucleus ventralis posterolateralis

26 Corpus geniculatum mediale
27 Globus pallidus
28 Commissura anterior
29 Putamen
30 Pedunculus cerebri
31 Tractus opticus
32 Limbus Giacomini
33 Gyrus uncinatus
34 Gyrus semilunaris
35 Ventriculus lateralis, cornu inferius
36 Cornu ammonis
37 Corpus amygdaloideum

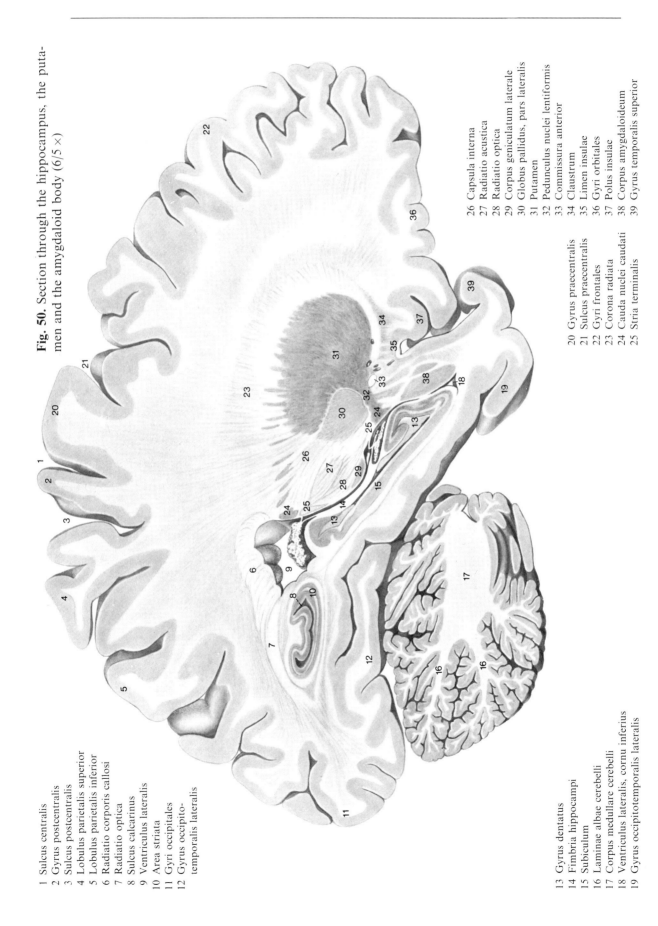

Fig. 50. Section through the hippocampus, the putamen and the amygdaloid body (6/5 ×)

1 Sulcus centralis
2 Gyrus postcentralis
3 Sulcus postcentralis
4 Lobulus parietalis superior
5 Lobulus parietalis inferior
6 Radiatio corporis callosi
7 Radiatio optica
8 Sulcus calcarinus
9 Ventriculus lateralis
10 Area striata
11 Gyri occipitales
12 Gyrus occipito-
temporalis lateralis

13 Gyrus dentatus
14 Fimbria hippocampi
15 Subiculum
16 Laminae albae cerebelli
17 Corpus medullare cerebelli
18 Ventriculus lateralis, cornu inferius
19 Gyrus occipitotemporalis lateralis

20 Gyrus praecentralis
21 Sulcus praecentralis
22 Gyri frontales
23 Corona radiata
24 Cauda nuclei caudati
25 Stria terminalis

26 Capsula interna
27 Radiatio acustica
28 Radiatio optica
29 Corpus geniculatum laterale
30 Globus pallidus, pars lateralis
31 Putamen
32 Pedunculus nuclei lentiformis
33 Commissura anterior
34 Claustrum
35 Limen insulae
36 Gyri orbitales
37 Polus insulae
38 Corpus amygdaloideum
39 Gyrus temporalis superior

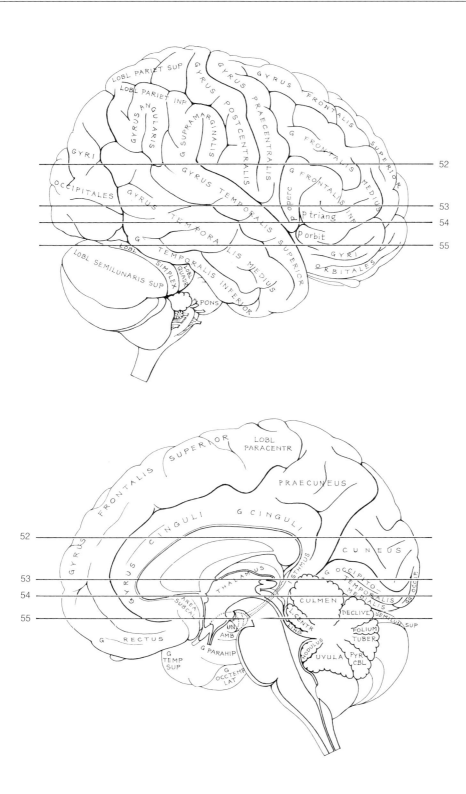

Fig. 51. Key diagrams showing the level and plane of the horizontal sections in Figures 52–55 (2/3×)

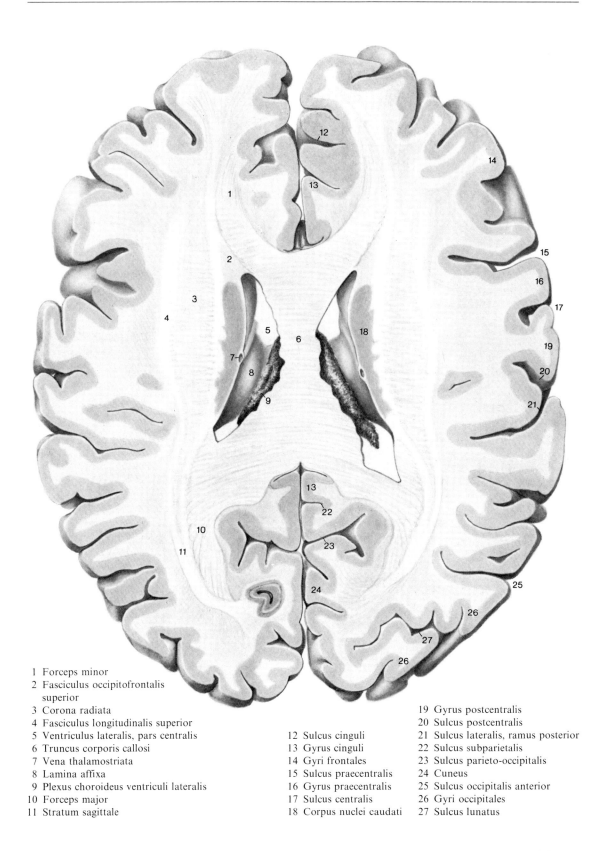

1 Forceps minor
2 Fasciculus occipitofrontalis
   superior
3 Corona radiata
4 Fasciculus longitudinalis superior
5 Ventriculus lateralis, pars centralis
6 Truncus corporis callosi
7 Vena thalamostriata
8 Lamina affixa
9 Plexus choroideus ventriculi lateralis
10 Forceps major
11 Stratum sagittale

12 Sulcus cinguli
13 Gyrus cinguli
14 Gyri frontales
15 Sulcus praecentralis
16 Gyrus praecentralis
17 Sulcus centralis
18 Corpus nuclei caudati

19 Gyrus postcentralis
20 Sulcus postcentralis
21 Sulcus lateralis, ramus posterior
22 Sulcus subparietalis
23 Sulcus parieto-occipitalis
24 Cuneus
25 Sulcus occipitalis anterior
26 Gyri occipitales
27 Sulcus lunatus

Fig. 52. Section through the corpus callosum and the body of the caudate nucleus. The thickness of this slice is twice the standard of 2 mm (6/5 ×)

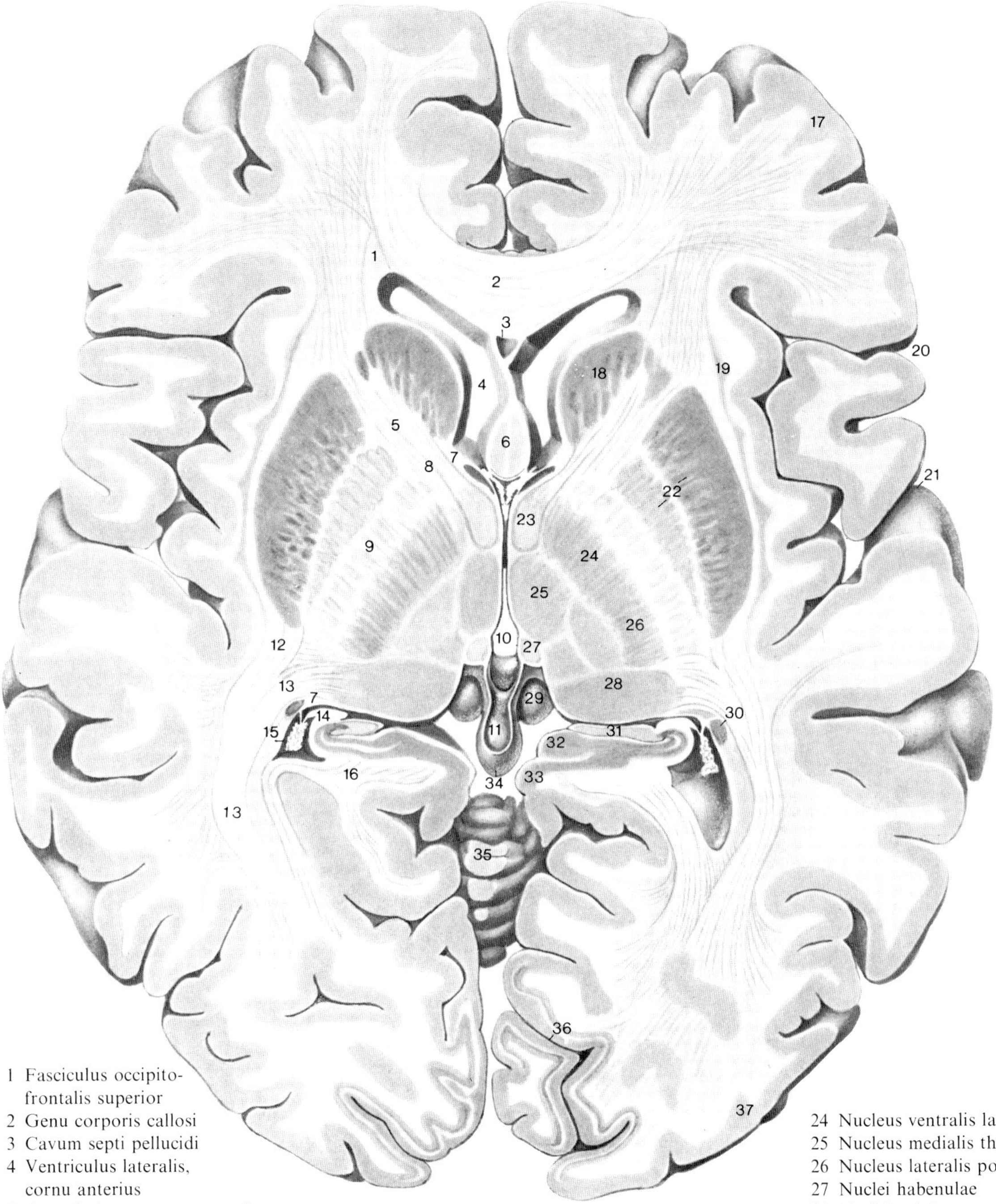

Fig. 53. Section through the striate body, the thalamus and the internal capsule. The thickness of this slice is twice the standard of 2 mm (6/5 ×)

1 Fasciculus occipito-
   frontalis superior
2 Genu corporis callosi
3 Cavum septi pellucidi
4 Ventriculus lateralis,
   cornu anterius
5 Capsula interna, crus anterius
6 Fornix
7 Stria terminalis
8 Capsula interna, genu
9 Capsula interna, crus posterius
10 Ventriculus tertius
11 Recessus suprapinealis
12 Fasciculus longitudinalis superior
13 Radiatio optica
14 Fimbria hippocampi

15 Ventriculus lateralis, cornu inferius
16 Radiatio corporis callosi
17 Gyri frontales
18 Caput nuclei caudati
19 Claustrum
20 Sulcus lateralis, ramus ascendens
21 Sulcus lateralis, ramus posterior
22 Nucleus lentiformis
23 Nucleus anterior thalami

24 Nucleus ventralis lateralis
25 Nucleus medialis thalami
26 Nucleus lateralis posterior
27 Nuclei habenulae
28 Nuclei pulvinares
29 Colliculus superior
30 Cauda nuclei caudati
31 Fasciola cinerea
32 Gyrus fasciolaris
33 Gyri Andreae Retzii
34 Corpus pineale
35 Vermis cerebelli
36 Sulcus calcarinus
37 Gyri occipitales

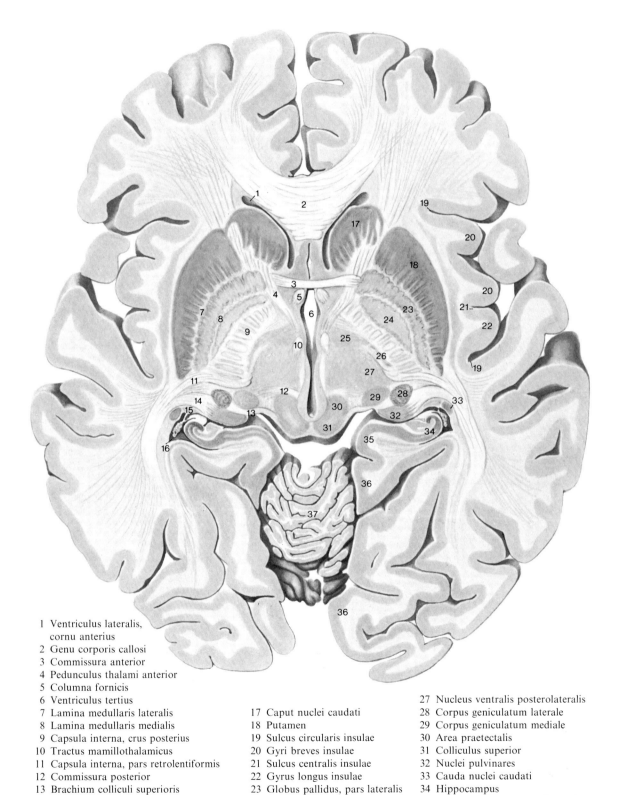

1 Ventriculus lateralis,
  cornu anterius
2 Genu corporis callosi
3 Commissura anterior
4 Pedunculus thalami anterior
5 Columna fornicis
6 Ventriculus tertius
7 Lamina medullaris lateralis   17 Caput nuclei caudati   27 Nucleus ventralis posterolateralis
8 Lamina medullaris medialis   18 Putamen   28 Corpus geniculatum laterale
9 Capsula interna, crus posterius   19 Sulcus circularis insulae   29 Corpus geniculatum mediale
10 Tractus mamillothalamicus   20 Gyri breves insulae   30 Area praetectalis
11 Capsula interna, pars retrolentiformis 21 Sulcus centralis insulae   31 Colliculus superior
12 Commissura posterior   22 Gyrus longus insulae   32 Nuclei pulvinares
13 Brachium colliculi superioris   23 Globus pallidus, pars lateralis   33 Cauda nuclei caudati
14 Radiatio optica   24 Globus pallidus, pars medialis   34 Hippocampus
15 Stria terminalis   25 Zona incerta   35 Gyrus parahippocampalis
16 Ventriculus lateralis, cornu inferius   26 Nucleus reticularis thalami   36 Gyrus occipitotemporalis medialis
                                                                             37 Lobus anterior cerebelli

Fig. 54. Section through the striate body, the anterior commissure and the superior colliculus
(6/5×)

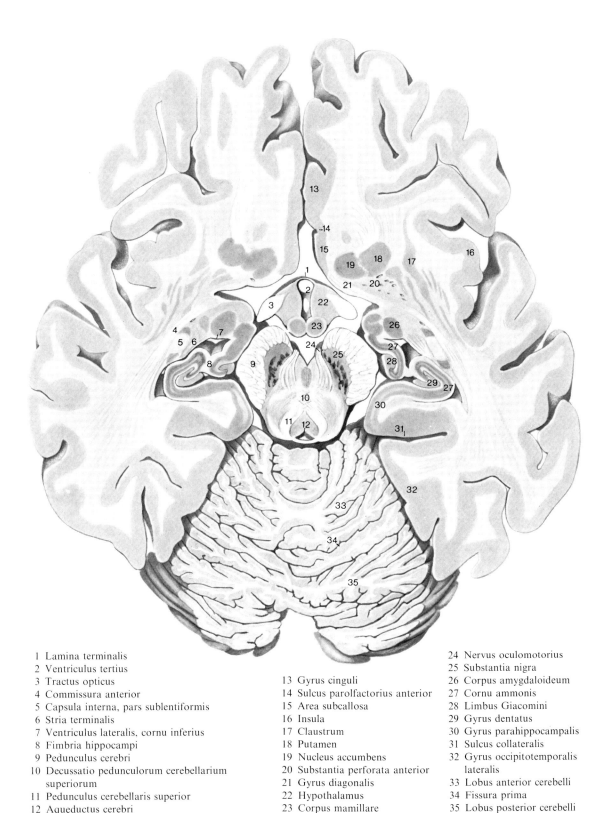

1 Lamina terminalis
2 Ventriculus tertius
3 Tractus opticus
4 Commissura anterior
5 Capsula interna, pars sublentiformis
6 Stria terminalis
7 Ventriculus lateralis, cornu inferius
8 Fimbria hippocampi
9 Pedunculus cerebri
10 Decussatio pedunculorum cerebellarium
   superiorum
11 Pedunculus cerebellaris superior
12 Aqueductus cerebri

13 Gyrus cinguli
14 Sulcus parolfactorius anterior
15 Area subcallosa
16 Insula
17 Claustrum
18 Putamen
19 Nucleus accumbens
20 Substantia perforata anterior
21 Gyrus diagonalis
22 Hypothalamus
23 Corpus mamillare

24 Nervus oculomotorius
25 Substantia nigra
26 Corpus amygdaloideum
27 Cornu ammonis
28 Limbus Giacomini
29 Gyrus dentatus
30 Gyrus parahippocampalis
31 Sulcus collateralis
32 Gyrus occipitotemporalis
   lateralis
33 Lobus anterior cerebelli
34 Fissura prima
35 Lobus posterior cerebelli

Fig. 55. Section through the mamillary body and the cerebral peduncle (6/5 ×)

Part III Microscopical Sections

Coronal Sections Through the Basal Part
of the Prosencephalon

Transverse Sections Through the Brain
Stem and Spinal Cord

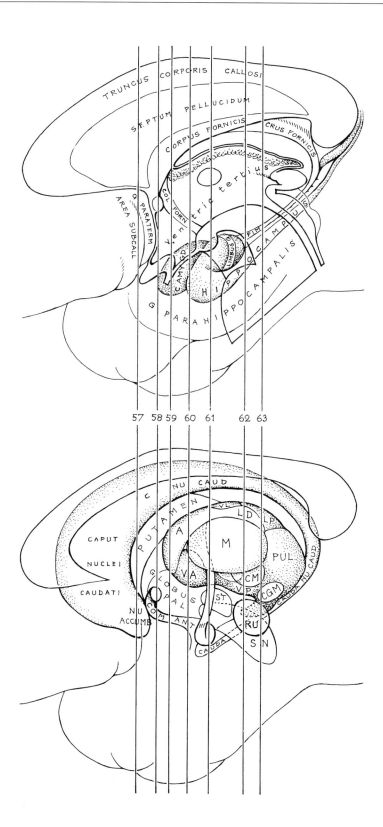

Fig. 56. Key diagrams showing level and plane of the sections illustrated in Figures 57–63. *Above*: medial view; *below*: deep structures exposed from the same side

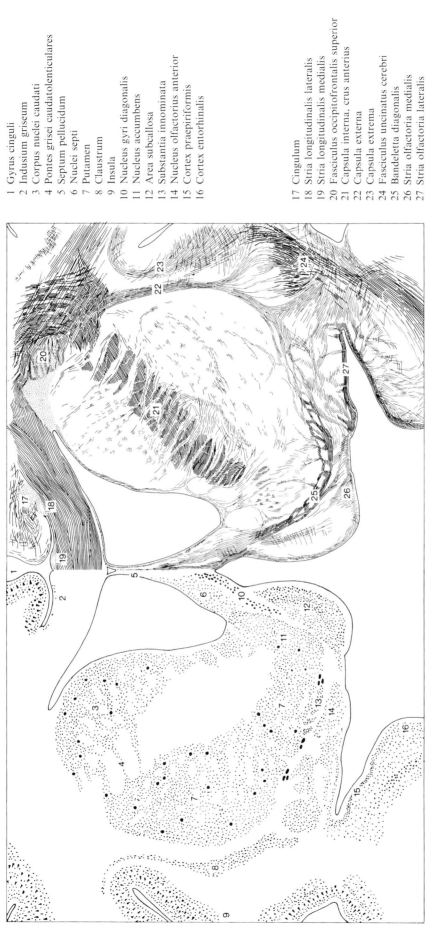

1 Gyrus cinguli
2 Indusium griseum
3 Corpus nuclei caudati
4 Pontes grisei caudatolenticulares
5 Septum pellucidum
6 Nuclei septi
7 Putamen
8 Claustrum
9 Insula
10 Nucleus gyri diagonalis
11 Nucleus accumbens
12 Area subcallosa
13 Substantia innominata
14 Nucleus olfactorius anterior
15 Cortex praepiriformis
16 Cortex entorhinalis

17 Cingulum
18 Stria longitudinalis lateralis
19 Stria longitudinalis medialis
20 Fasciculus occipitofrontalis superior
21 Capsula interna, crus anterius
22 Capsula externa
23 Capsula extrema
24 Fasciculus uncinatus cerebri
25 Bandeletta diagonalis
26 Stria olfactoria medialis
27 Stria olfactoria lateralis

Fig. 57. Section through the septal area (5/2 ×)

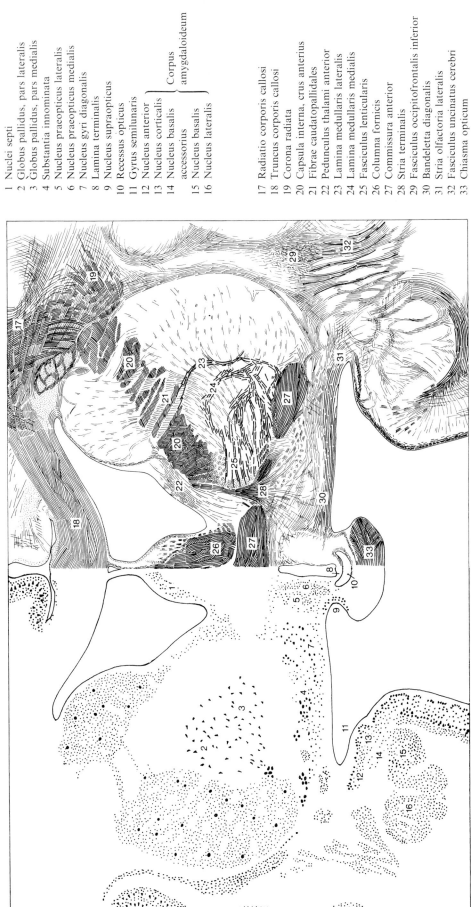

1 Nuclei septi
2 Globus pallidus, pars lateralis
3 Globus pallidus, pars medialis
4 Substantia innominata
5 Nucleus praeopticus lateralis
6 Nucleus praeopticus medialis
7 Nucleus gyri diagonalis
8 Lamina terminalis
9 Nucleus supraopticus
10 Recessus opticus
11 Gyrus semilunaris
12 Nucleus anterior
13 Nucleus corticalis
14 Nucleus basalis
   accessorius
15 Nucleus basalis
16 Nucleus lateralis
⎫
⎬ Corpus
⎭ amygdaloideum

17 Radiatio corporis callosi
18 Truncus corporis callosi
19 Corona radiata
20 Capsula interna, crus anterius
21 Fibrae caudatopallidales
22 Pedunculus thalami anterior
23 Lamina medullaris lateralis
24 Lamina medullaris medialis
25 Fasciculus lenticularis
26 Columna fornicis
27 Commissura anterior
28 Stria terminalis
29 Fasciculus occipitofrontalis inferior
30 Bandeletta diagonalis
31 Stria olfactoria lateralis
32 Fasciculus uncinatus cerebri
33 Chiasma opticum

Fig. 58. Section through the anterior commissure and the optic chiasm (5/2 ×)

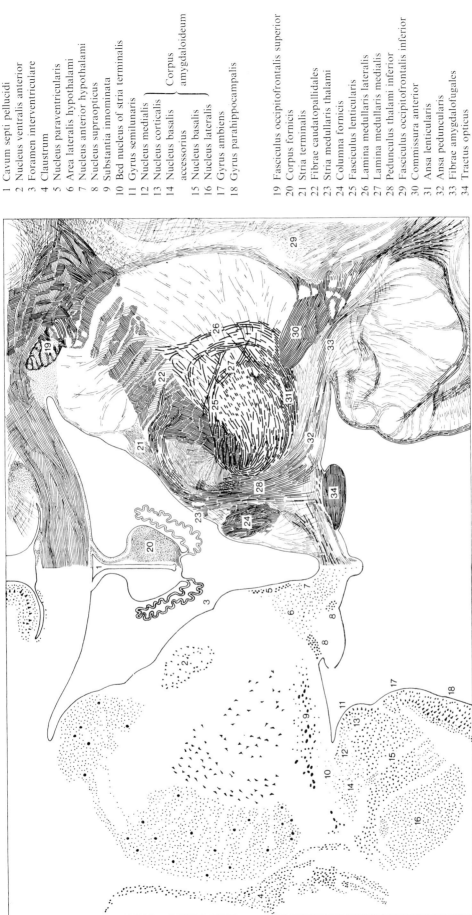

1 Cavum septi pellucidi
2 Nucleus ventralis anterior
3 Foramen interventriculare
4 Claustrum
5 Nucleus paraventricularis
6 Area lateralis hypothalami
7 Nucleus anterior hypothalami
8 Nucleus supraopticus
9 Substantia innominata
10 Bed nucleus of stria terminalis
11 Gyrus semilunaris
12 Nucleus medialis
13 Nucleus corticalis
14 Nucleus basalis   ⎫
   accessorius   ⎬ Corpus
15 Nucleus basalis   ⎪ amygdaloideum
16 Nucleus lateralis   ⎭
17 Gyrus ambiens
18 Gyrus parahippocampalis

19 Fasciculus occipitofrontalis superior
20 Corpus fornicis
21 Stria terminalis
22 Fibrae caudatopallidales
23 Stria medullaris thalami
24 Columna fornicis
25 Fasciculus lenticularis
26 Lamina medullaris lateralis
27 Lamina medullaris medialis
28 Pedunculus thalami inferior
29 Fasciculus occipitofrontalis inferior
30 Commissura anterior
31 Ansa lenticularis
32 Ansa peduncularis
33 Fibrae amygdalofugales
34 Tractus opticus

Fig. 59. Section through the interventricular foramen, the hypothalamus and the amygdaloid body (5/2 ×)

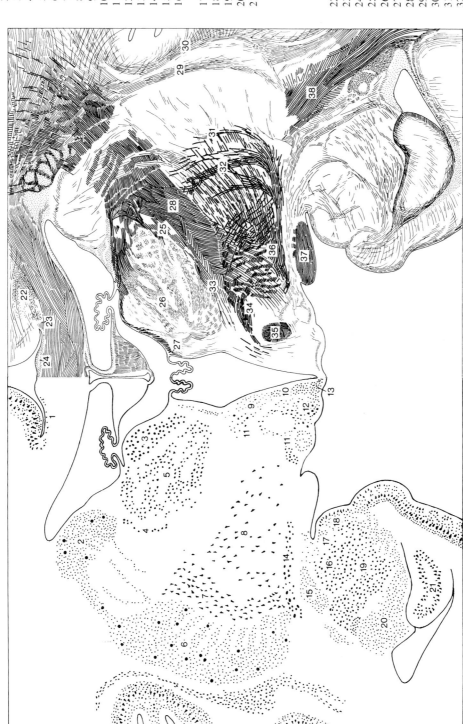

1 Indusium griseum
2 Corpus nuclei caudati
3 Nucleus anterior thalami
4 Nucleus reticularis thalami
5 Nucleus ventralis anterior
6 Putamen
7 Globus pallidus, pars lateralis
8 Globus pallidus, pars medialis
9 Nucleus posterior hypothalami
10 Nucleus ventromedialis
11 Area lateralis hypothalami
12 Nuclei tuberales
13 Nucleus infundibularis
14 Substantia innominata
15 Nucleus centralis
16 Nucleus basalis accessorius
17 Nucleus medialis
18 Nucleus corticalis
19 Nucleus basalis
20 Nucleus lateralis
21 Cornu ammonis

} Corpus amygdaloideum

22 Cingulum
23 Stria longitudinalis lateralis
24 Stria longitudinalis medialis
25 Lamina medullaris externa
26 Lamina medullaris interna
27 Stria medullaris thalami
28 Capsula interna, crus posterius
29 Capsula externa
30 Capsula extrema
31 Lamina medullaris lateralis
32 Lamina medullaris medialis
33 Fasciculus thalamicus
34 Fasciculus lenticularis
35 Columna fornicis
36 Ansa lenticularis
37 Tractus opticus
38 Commissura anterior

Fig. 60. Section through the rostral part of the thalamus, the amygdaloid body and the rostral pole of the hippocampus (5/2 ×)

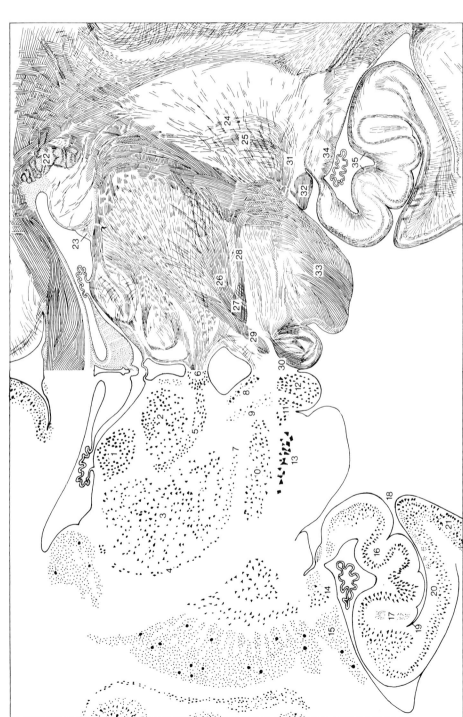

1 Nucleus anterior thalami
2 Nucleus medialis thalami
3 Nucleus ventralis lateralis
4 Nucleus reticularis thalami
5 Nuclei intralaminares
6 Nuclei mediani thalami
7 Zona incerta
8 Nucleus posterior hypothalami
9 Area lateralis hypothalami
10 Nucleus subthalamicus
11 Corpus mamillare, nucleus lateralis
12 Corpus mamillare, nucleus medialis
13 Substantia nigra
14 Corpus amygdaloideum,
    nucleus basalis accessorius
15 Pedunculus nuclei lentiformis
16 Cornu ammonis
17 Fascia dentata
18 Incisura unci
19 Sulcus hippocampi
20 Subiculum
21 Cortex entorhinalis

22 Fasciculus occipitofrontalis
    superior
23 Stria terminalis (1)
24 Lamina medullaris lateralis
25 Lamina medullaris medialis
26 Fasciculus thalamicus
27 Area tegmentalis H
28 Fasciculus lenticularis
29 Tractus mamillothalamicus
30 Fasciculus mamillaris princeps
31 Ansa lenticularis
32 Tractus opticus
33 Pedunculus cerebri
34 Stria terminalis (2)
35 Alveus hippocampi

Fig. 61. Section through the centre of the third ventricle, the mamillary body and the hippocampus (5/2 ×)

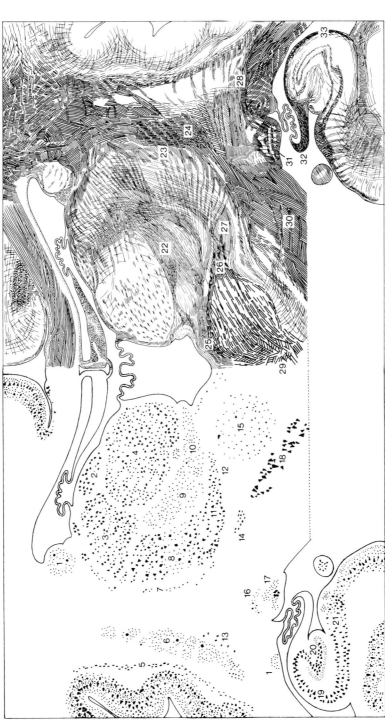

1 Cauda nuclei caudati
2 Nucleus lateralis dorsalis
3 Nucleus lateralis posterior
4 Nucleus medialis thalami
5 Claustrum
6 Putamen
7 Nucleus reticularis thalami
8 Nucleus ventralis posterolateralis
9 Nucleus centromedianus
10 Nucleus parafascicularis
11 Nucleus ventralis posteromedialis
12 Nucleus ventralis posteromedialis, pars parvocellularis
13 Globus pallidus, pars lateralis
14 Zona incerta
15 Nucleus ruber
16 Nucleus praegeniculatus
17 Corpus geniculatum laterale
18 Substantia nigra
19 Cornu ammonis
20 Fascia dentata
21 Subiculum

22 Lamina medullaris interna
23 Lamina medullaris externa
24 Capsula interna, crus posterius
25 Fasciculus longitudinalis medialis
26 Pedunculus cerebellaris superior
27 Lemniscus medialis
28 Capsula interna, pars sublentiformis
29 Decussatio pedunculorum cerebellarium superiorum
30 Pedunculus cerebri
31 Tractus opticus
32 Fimbria hippocampi
33 Alveus hippocampi

Fig. 62. Section through the thalamus and the caudal end of the putamen (5/2 ×)

1 Gyrus cinguli
2 Indusium griseum
3 Cauda nuclei caudati
4 Nucleus lateralis dorsalis
5 Nucleus reticularis thalami
6 Nucleus lateralis posterior
7 Nucleus medialis thalami
8 Nuclei habenulae
9 Nucleus centromedianus
10 Nucleus ventralis posterolateralis
11 Pontes grisei caudatolenticulares
12 Nucleus interstitialis
13 Nucleus accessorius nervi
   oculomotorii
14 Substantia nigra
15 Corpus geniculatum mediale
16 Corpus geniculatum laterale
17 Cornu ammonis
18 Fascia dentata
19 Subiculum
20 Cortex entorhinalis

21 Cingulum
22 Stria longitudinalis lateralis
23 Stria longitudinalis medialis
24 Stria terminalis (1)
25 Crus fornicis
26 Stria medullaris thalami
27 Capsula interna,
   pars retrolentiformis
28 Tractus habenulointerpeduncularis
29 Fasciculus longitudinalis dorsalis
30 Fasciculus longitudinalis medialis
31 Pedunculus cerebellaris superior
32 Radiatio optica
33 Stria terminalis (2)
34 Fimbria hippocampi
35 Decussatio pedunculorum
   cerebellarium superiorum
36 Lemniscus medialis
37 Pedunculus cerebri

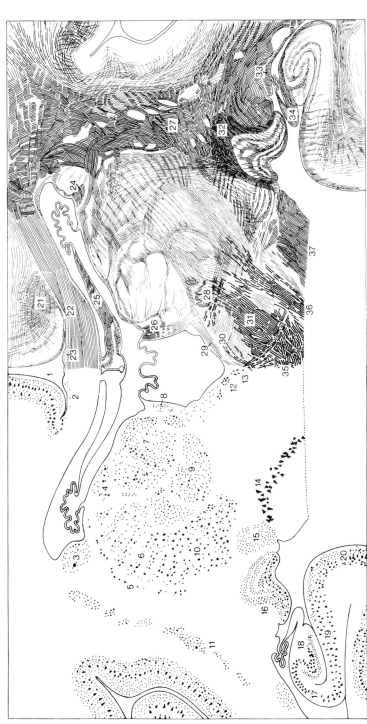

Fig. 63. Section through the medial and lateral geniculate bodies (5/2 ×)

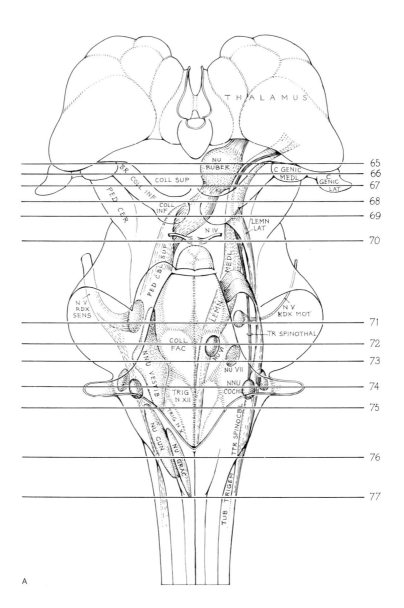

THALAMUS

NU RUBER

BR COLL INF

COLL SUP

PED CER

COLL INF

C GENIC MEDL

C GENIC LAT

LEMN LAT

N IV

PED CBL SUP

LEMN MEDL

N V RDX SENS

N V RDX MOT

TR SPINOTHAL

COLL FAC

NU VI

NNU VESTIB

NU VII

NNU COCHL

TRIG N XII

TRIG N X

TR SPINOCBL

NU CUN

NU GRAC

TUB TRIGEM

65
66
67
68
69
70
71
72
73
74
75
76
77

A

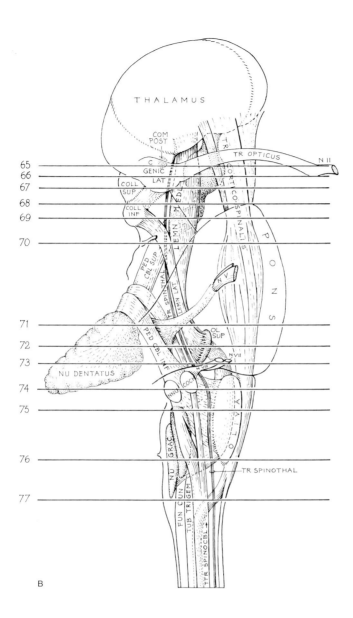

Fig. 64A and B. Key diagrams showing level and plane of the sections illustrated in Figures 65–77. *Left*: dorsal view; *right*: lateral view

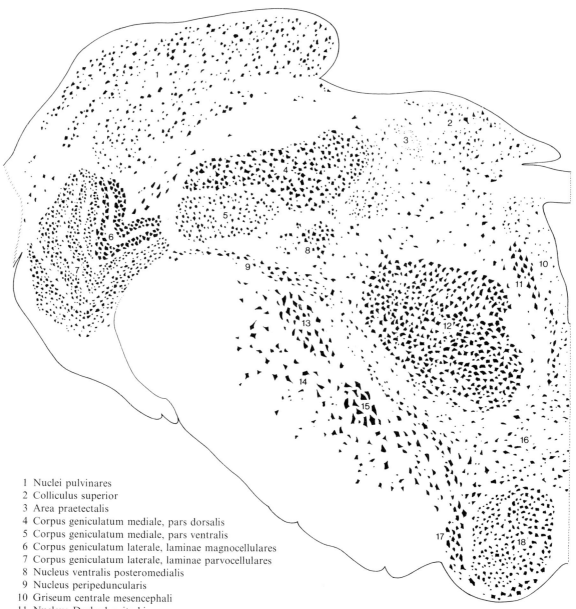

1 Nuclei pulvinares
2 Colliculus superior
3 Area praetectalis
4 Corpus geniculatum mediale, pars dorsalis
5 Corpus geniculatum mediale, pars ventralis
6 Corpus geniculatum laterale, laminae magnocellulares
7 Corpus geniculatum laterale, laminae parvocellulares
8 Nucleus ventralis posteromedialis
9 Nucleus peripeduncularis
10 Griseum centrale mesencephali
11 Nucleus Darkschewitschi
12 Nucleus ruber, pars parvocellularis
13 Nucleus subthalamicus
14 Substantia nigra, pars reticulata
15 Substantia nigra, pars compacta
16 Area tegmentalis ventralis
17 Corpus mamillare, nucleus lateralis
18 Corpus mamillare, nucleus medialis

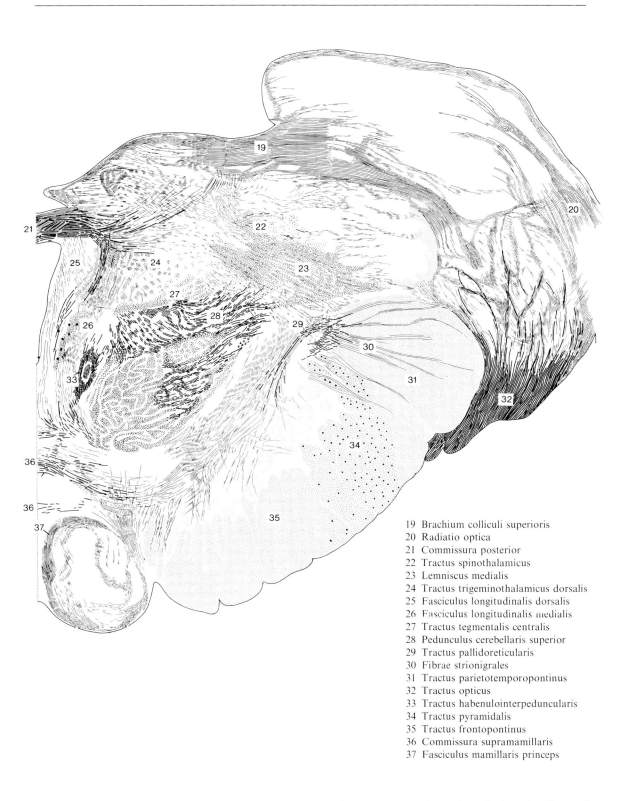

19 Brachium colliculi superioris
20 Radiatio optica
21 Commissura posterior
22 Tractus spinothalamicus
23 Lemniscus medialis
24 Tractus trigeminothalamicus dorsalis
25 Fasciculus longitudinalis dorsalis
26 Fasciculus longitudinalis medialis
27 Tractus tegmentalis centralis
28 Pedunculus cerebellaris superior
29 Tractus pallidoreticularis
30 Fibrae strionigrales
31 Tractus parietotemporopontinus
32 Tractus opticus
33 Tractus habenulointerpeduncularis
34 Tractus pyramidalis
35 Tractus frontopontinus
36 Commissura supramamillaris
37 Fasciculus mamillaris princeps

Fig. 65. Section through the posterior commissure, the medial and lateral geniculate bodies and the mamillary body (7/1 ×)

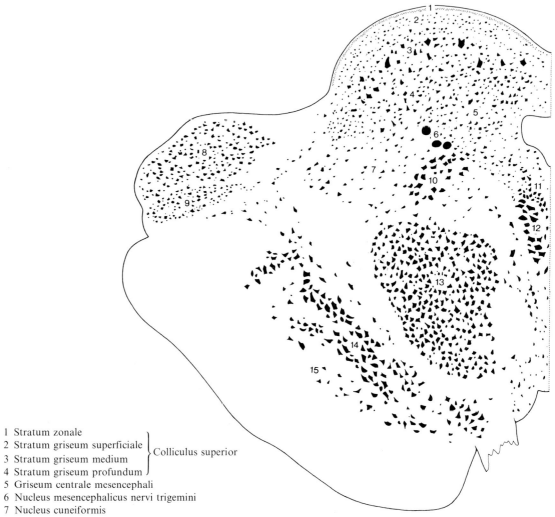

1 Stratum zonale
2 Stratum griseum superficiale ⎫
3 Stratum griseum medium   ⎬ Colliculus superior
4 Stratum griseum profundum   ⎭
5 Griseum centrale mesencephali
6 Nucleus mesencephalicus nervi trigemini
7 Nucleus cuneiformis
8 Corpus geniculatum mediale, pars dorsalis
9 Corpus geniculatum mediale, pars ventralis
10 Nucleus interstitialis
11 Nucleus accessorius nervi oculomotorii
12 Nucleus nervi oculomotorii
13 Nucleus ruber, pars parvocellularis
14 Substantia nigra, pars compacta
15 Substantia nigra, pars reticulata

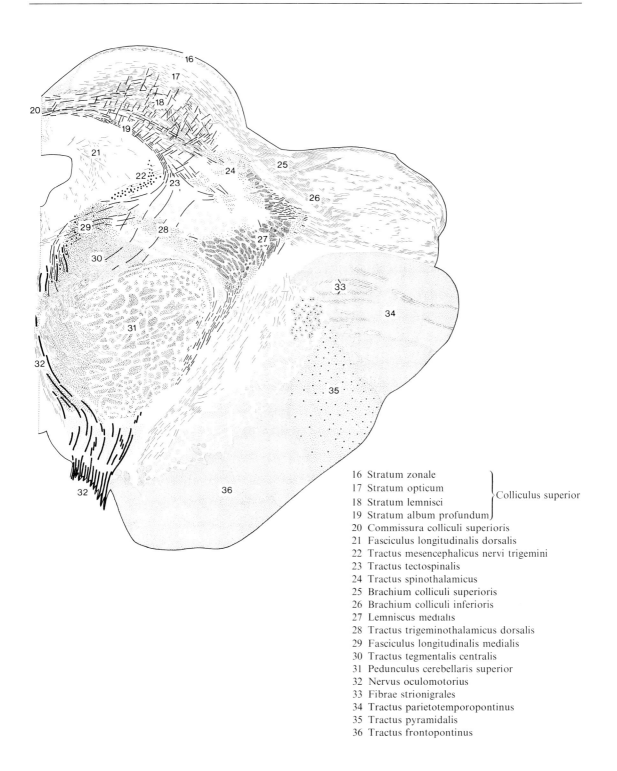

16 Stratum zonale
17 Stratum opticum   ⎫
18 Stratum lemnisci   ⎬ Colliculus superior
19 Stratum album profundum   ⎭
20 Commissura colliculi superioris
21 Fasciculus longitudinalis dorsalis
22 Tractus mesencephalicus nervi trigemini
23 Tractus tectospinalis
24 Tractus spinothalamicus
25 Brachium colliculi superioris
26 Brachium colliculi inferioris
27 Lemniscus medialis
28 Tractus trigeminothalamicus dorsalis
29 Fasciculus longitudinalis medialis
30 Tractus tegmentalis centralis
31 Pedunculus cerebellaris superior
32 Nervus oculomotorius
33 Fibrae strionigrales
34 Tractus parietotemporopontinus
35 Tractus pyramidalis
36 Tractus frontopontinus

Fig. 66. Section through the red nucleus and the medial geniculate body (7/1 ×)

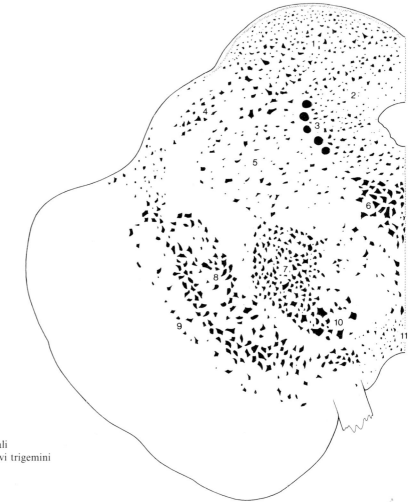

 1 Colliculus superior
 2 Griseum centrale mesencephali
 3 Nucleus mesencephalicus nervi trigemini
 4 Nucleus paralemniscalis
 5 Nucleus cuneiformis
 6 Nucleus nervi oculomotorii
 7 Nucleus ruber, pars parvocellularis
 8 Substantia nigra, pars compacta
 9 Substantia nigra, pars reticulata
10 Nucleus ruber, pars magnocellularis
11 Nucleus interpeduncularis

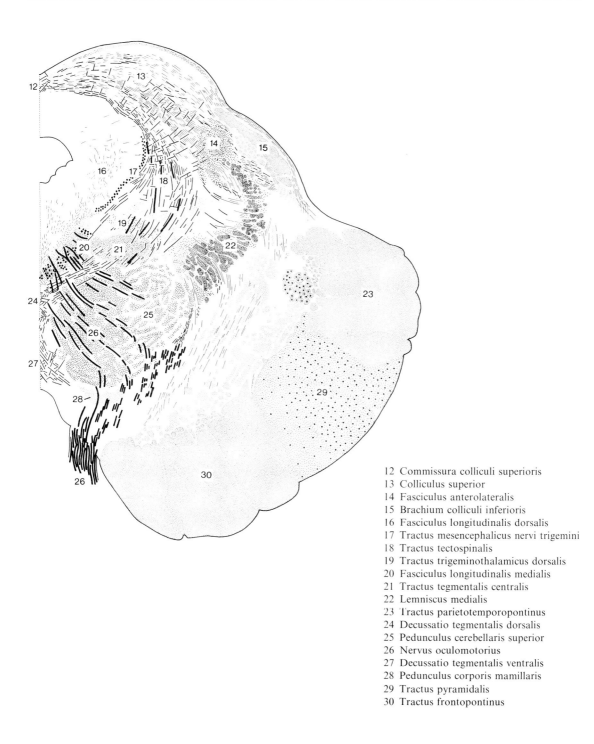

12 Commissura colliculi superioris
13 Colliculus superior
14 Fasciculus anterolateralis
15 Brachium colliculi inferioris
16 Fasciculus longitudinalis dorsalis
17 Tractus mesencephalicus nervi trigemini
18 Tractus tectospinalis
19 Tractus trigeminothalamicus dorsalis
20 Fasciculus longitudinalis medialis
21 Tractus tegmentalis centralis
22 Lemniscus medialis
23 Tractus parietotemporopontinus
24 Decussatio tegmentalis dorsalis
25 Pedunculus cerebellaris superior
26 Nervus oculomotorius
27 Decussatio tegmentalis ventralis
28 Pedunculus corporis mamillaris
29 Tractus pyramidalis
30 Tractus frontopontinus

Fig. 67. Section through the superior colliculus and the oculomotor nuclei (7/1 ×)

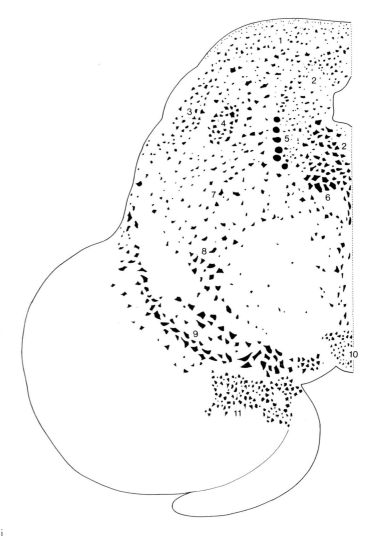

1 Nucleus intercollicularis
2 Griseum centrale mesencephali
3 Nucleus paralemniscalis
4 Nucleus centralis colliculi inferioris
5 Nucleus mesencephalicus nervi trigemini
6 Nucleus nervi trochlearis
7 Nucleus cuneiformis
8 Nucleus tegmentalis pedunculopontinus, pars dissipata
9 Substantia nigra, pars compacta
10 Nucleus interpeduncularis
11 Nuclei pontis

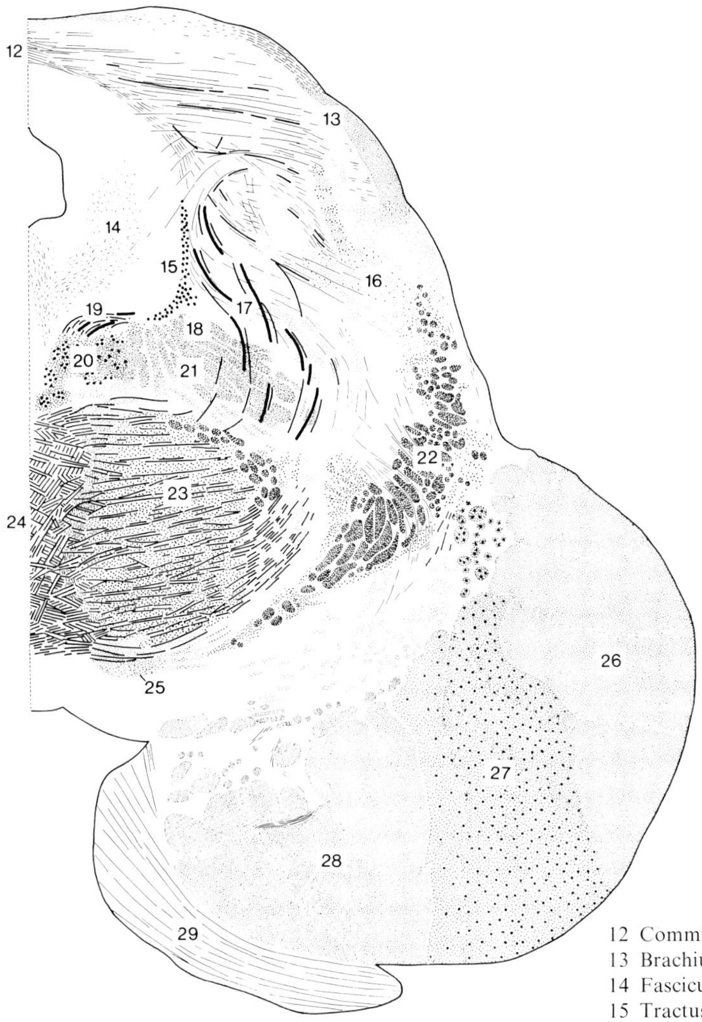

Fig. 68. Section through the intercollicular area and the trochlear nucleus (7/1 ×)

12 Commissura colliculi inferioris
13 Brachium colliculi inferioris
14 Fasciculus longitudinalis dorsalis
15 Tractus mesencephalicus nervi trigemini
16 Fasciculus anterolateralis
17 Tractus tectospinalis
18 Tractus trigeminothalamicus dorsalis
19 Nervus trochlearis
20 Fasciculus longitudinalis medialis
21 Tractus tegmentalis centralis
22 Lemniscus medialis
23 Pedunculus cerebellaris superior
24 Decussatio pedunculorum cerebellarium superiorum
25 Pedunculus mamillaris
26 Tractus parietotemporopontinus
27 Tractus pyramidalis
28 Tractus frontopontinus
29 Fibrae pontocerebellares

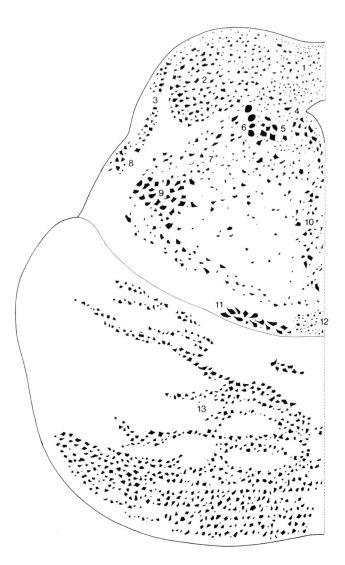

1 Nucleus intercollicularis
2 Colliculus inferior, nucleus centralis
3 Colliculus inferior, zona lateralis
4 Griseum centrale mesencephali
5 Locus coeruleus
6 Nucleus mesencephalicus nervi trigemini
7 Nucleus cuneiformis
8 Corpus parabigeminum
9 Nucleus tegmentalis pedunculopontinus,
  pars compacta
10 Nucleus centralis superior
11 Substantia nigra, pars compacta
12 Nucleus interpeduncularis
13 Nuclei pontis

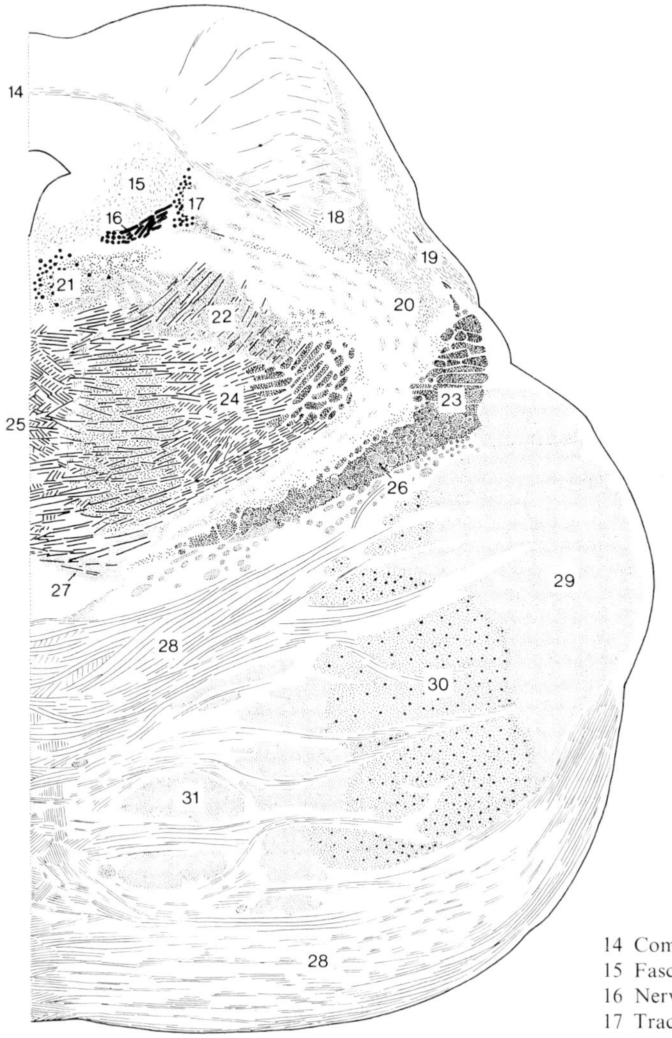

14 Commissura colliculi inferioris
15 Fasciculus longitudinalis dorsalis
16 Nervus trochlearis
17 Tractus mesencephalicus nervi trigemini
18 Lemniscus lateralis
19 Tractus tectopontinus
20 Fasciculus anterolateralis
21 Fasciculus longitudinalis medialis
22 Tractus tegmentalis centralis
23 Lemniscus medialis
24 Pedunculus cerebellaris superior
25 Decussatio pedunculorum cerebellarium superiorum
26 Fibrae corticotegmentales
27 Pedunculus mamillaris
28 Fibrae pontocerebellares
29 Tractus parietotemporopontinus
30 Tractus pyramidalis
31 Tractus frontopontinus

Fig. 69. Section through the inferior colliculus and the decussation of the superior cerebellar peduncles (7/1 ×)

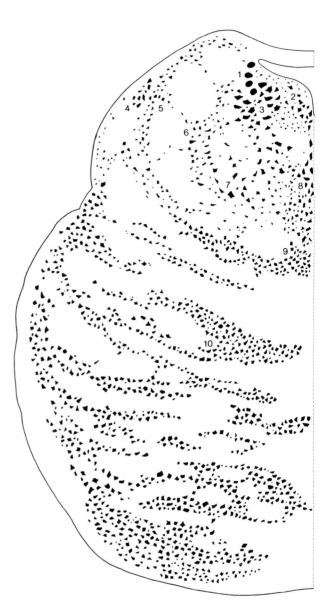

1 Nucleus mesencephalicus nervi trigemini
2 Griseum centrale mesencephali
3 Locus coeruleus
4 Nucleus lemnisci lateralis
5 Nucleus parabrachialis lateralis
6 Nucleus parabrachialis medialis
7 Nucleus reticularis pontis oralis
8 Nucleus centralis superior
9 Nucleus reticularis tegmenti pontis
10 Nuclei pontis

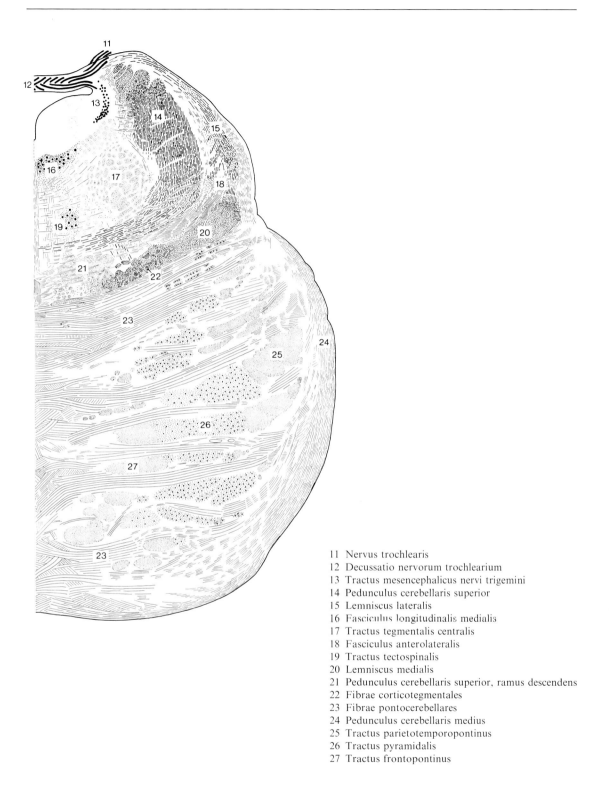

11 Nervus trochlearis
12 Decussatio nervorum trochlearium
13 Tractus mesencephalicus nervi trigemini
14 Pedunculus cerebellaris superior
15 Lemniscus lateralis
16 Fasciculus longitudinalis medialis
17 Tractus tegmentalis centralis
18 Fasciculus anterolateralis
19 Tractus tectospinalis
20 Lemniscus medialis
21 Pedunculus cerebellaris superior, ramus descendens
22 Fibrae corticotegmentales
23 Fibrae pontocerebellares
24 Pedunculus cerebellaris medius
25 Tractus parietotemporopontinus
26 Tractus pyramidalis
27 Tractus frontopontinus

Fig. 70. Section through the decussation of the trochlear nerves (7/1 ×)

1 Nucleus dentatus
2 Nucleus emboliformis
3 Nucleus globosus
4 Nucleus fastigii
5 Nucleus vestibularis superior
6 Griseum centrale metencephali
7 Nucleus mesencephalicus nervi trigemini
8 Nucleus sensorius principalis nervi trigemini
9 Nucleus motorius nervi trigemini
10 Nucleus reticularis pontis caudalis
11 Formatio reticularis lateralis
12 Nucleus lemnisci lateralis
13 Nucleus raphes pontis
14 Nucleus reticularis tegmenti pontis
15 Nuclei pontis

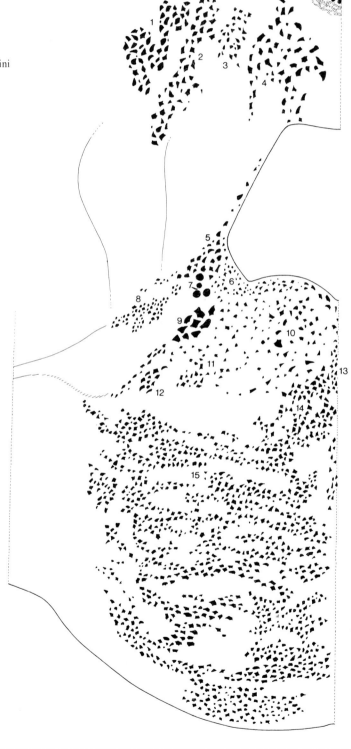

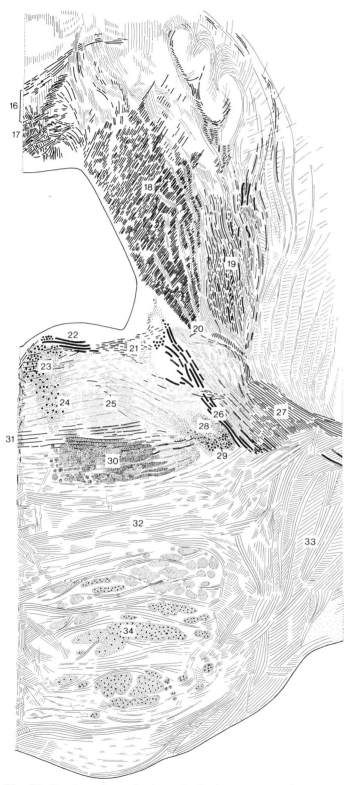

16 Commissura cerebelli
17 Decussatio fasciculorum uncinatorum
   cerebelli
18 Pedunculus cerebellaris superior
19 Pedunculus cerebellaris inferior
20 Fasciculus ovalis
21 Tractus vestibulomesencephalicus
22 Genu nervi facialis
23 Fasciculus longitudinalis medialis
24 Tractus tectospinalis
25 Tractus tegmentalis centralis
26 Nervus trigeminus, radix motoria
27 Nervus trigeminus, radix sensoria
28 Lemniscus lateralis
29 Fasciculus anterolateralis
30 Lemniscus medialis
31 Decussatio tractuum trigemino-
   thalamicorum ventralium
32 Fibrae pontocerebellares
33 Pedunculus cerebellaris medius
34 Tractus pyramidalis

Fig. 71. Section through the principal sensory and motor nuclei of the trigeminal nerve (7/1 ×)

1 Nucleus dentatus
2 Nucleus emboliformis
3 Nucleus globosus
4 Nucleus fastigii
5 Nucleus vestibularis superior
6 Nucleus vestibularis lateralis
7 Nucleus vestibularis medialis
8 Nucleus nervi abducentis
9 Formatio reticularis lateralis
10 Nucleus sensorius principalis nervi trigemini
11 Nucleus nervi facialis
12 Nucleus gigantocellularis
13 Nucleus raphes magnus
14 Nucleus lateralis olivae superioris
15 Nucleus medialis olivae superioris
16 Nucleus corporis trapezoidei
17 Nuclei pontis

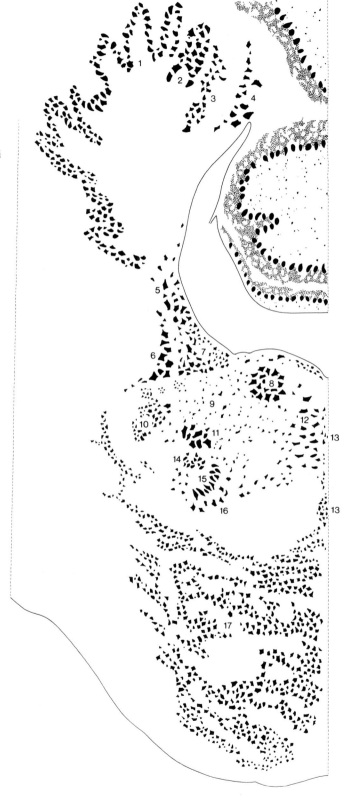

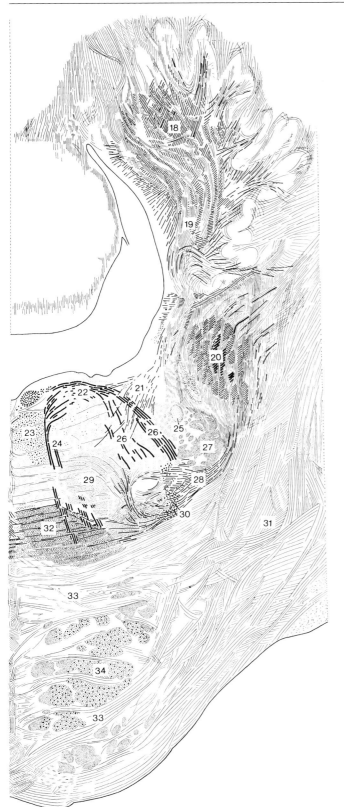

18 Pedunculus cerebellaris superior
19 Fibrae cerebellovestibulares
20 Pedunculus cerebellaris inferior
21 Tractus vestibulomesencephalicus + tractus
   vestibulospinalis
22 Genu nervi facialis
23 Fasciculus longitudinalis medialis
24 Nervus abducens
25 Fasciculus ovalis
26 Nervus facialis
27 Tractus spinalis nervi trigemini
28 Corpus trapezoideum
29 Tractus tegmentalis centralis
30 Fasciculus anterolateralis
31 Pedunculus cerebellaris medius
32 Lemniscus medialis + corpus trapezoideum
33 Fibrae pontocerebellares
34 Tractus pyramidalis

Fig. 72. Section through the abducens nucleus, the superior olive and the trapezoid body (7/1 ×)

1 Nucleus dentatus
2 Nucleus globosus
3 Nucleus vestibularis lateralis
4 Nucleus vestibularis medialis
5 Nucleus vestibularis inferior
6 Nucleus praepositus hypoglossi
7 Nucleus ovalis
8 Formatio reticularis lateralis
9 Nucleus spinalis nervi trigemini,
   pars oralis
10 Nucleus nervi facialis
11 Nucleus gigantocellularis
12 Nucleus raphes magnus
13 Oliva superior
14 Nucleus corporis trapezoidei
15 Corpus pontobulbare
16 Nuclei pontis

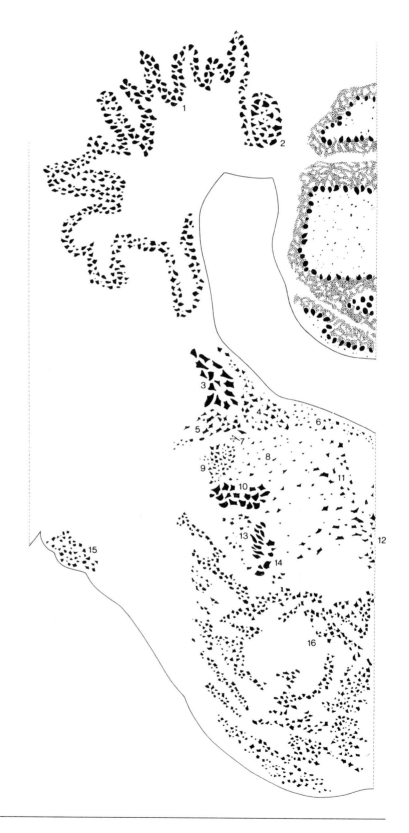

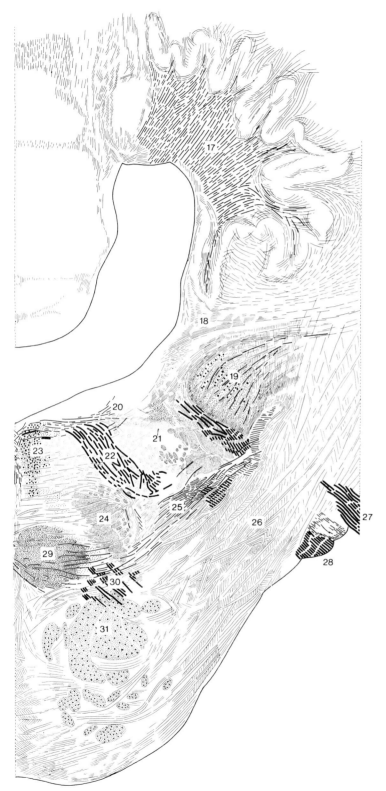

17 Pedunculus cerebellaris superior
18 Pedunculus flocculi
19 Pedunculus cerebellaris inferior
20 Tractus vestibulomesencephalicus +
   tractus vestibulo-spinalis
21 Fasciculus ovalis
22 Fibrae nervi facialis
23 Fasciculus longitudinalis medialis
24 Tractus tegmentalis centralis
25 Corpus trapezoideum
26 Pedunculus cerebellaris medius
27 Nervus vestibulocochlearis
28 Nervus facialis
29 Lemniscus medialis
30 Nervus abducens
31 Tractus pyramidalis

Fig. 73. Section through the vestibular nuclei and the motor nucleus of the facial nerve (7/1 ×)

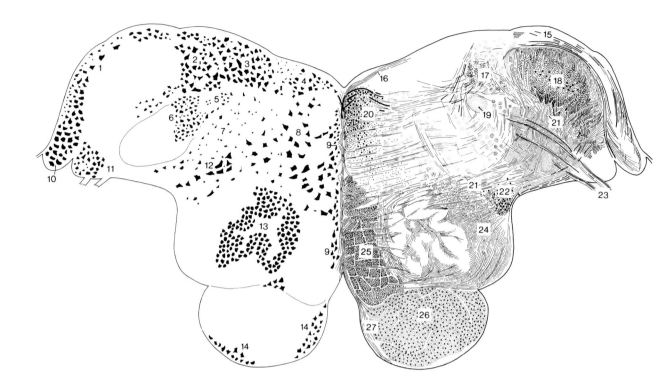

1 Nucleus cochlearis dorsalis
2 Nucleus vestibularis inferior
3 Nucleus vestibularis medialis
4 Nucleus praepositus hypoglossi
5 Nucleus solitarius
6 Nucleus spinalis nervi trigemini, pars oralis
7 Formatio reticularis lateralis
8 Nucleus gigantocellularis
9 Nucleus raphes magnus
10 Nucleus cochlearis ventralis
11 Corpus pontobulbare
12 Nucleus ambiguus
13 Nucleus olivaris inferior
14 Nuclei arcuati

15 Striae acusticae dorsales
16 Stria medullares ventriculi quarti
17 Nervus vestibularis, ramus descendens
18 Pedunculus cerebellaris inferior
19 Tractus solitarius
20 Fasciculus longitudinalis medialis
21 Fibrae olivocerebellares
22 Fasciculus anterolateralis
23 Nervus glossopharyngeus
24 Tractus tegmentalis centralis
25 Lemniscus medialis
26 Tractus pyramidalis
27 Fibrae arcuatae externae

Fig. 74. Section through the cochlear nuclei (7/1 ×)

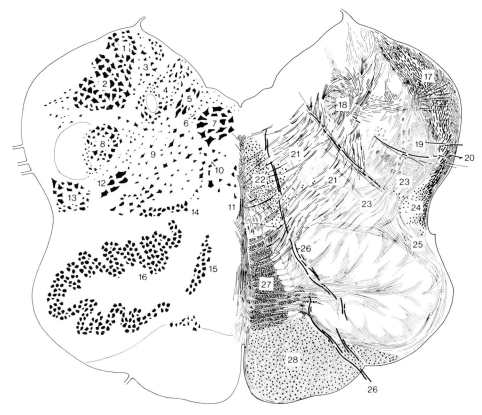

1 Nucleus cuneatus medialis
2 Nucleus cuneatus lateralis
3 Nucleus vestibularis inferior
4 Nucleus solitarius
5 Nucleus dorsalis nervi vagi
6 Nucleus intercalatus
7 Nucleus nervi hypoglossi
8 Nucleus spinalis nervi trigemini, pars interpolaris
9 Nucleus medullae oblongatae centralis
10 Nucleus funiculi anterioris
11 Nucleus raphes obscurus
12 Nucleus ambiguus
13 Nucleus funiculi lateralis
14 Nucleus olivaris accessorius dorsalis
15 Nucleus olivaris accessorius medialis
16 Nucleus olivaris inferior

17 Pedunculus cerebellaris inferior
18 Tractus solitarius
19 Tractus spinalis nervi trigemini
20 Nervus vagus
21 Fibrae arcuatae internae
22 Fasciculus longitudinalis medialis
23 Fibrae olivocerebellares
24 Fasciculus anterolateralis
25 Amiculum olivae
26 Nervus hypoglossus
27 Lemniscus medialis
28 Tractus pyramidalis

Fig. 75. Section through the middle part of the inferior olive (7/1 ×)

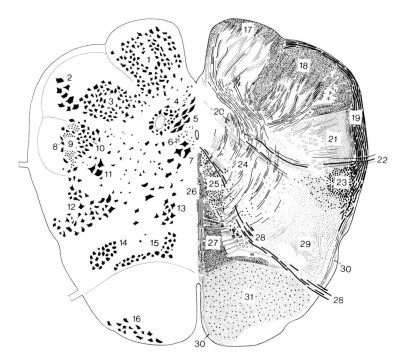

1 Nucleus gracilis
2 Nucleus cuneatus lateralis
3 Nucleus cuneatus medialis
4 Nucleus solitarius
5 Nucleus dorsalis nervi vagi
6 Nucleus intercalatus
7 Nucleus nervi hypoglossi
8 Cellulae marginales ⎫ Nucleus spinalis
9 Substantia gelatinosa ⎬ nervi trigemini,
10 Nucleus proprius ⎭ pars caudalis
11 Nucleus ambiguus
12 Nucleus funiculi lateralis
13 Nucleus funiculi anterioris
14 Nucleus olivaris inferior
15 Nucleus olivaris accessorius medialis
16 Nuclei arcuati

17 Fasciculus gracilis
18 Fasciculus cuneatus
19 Pedunculus cerebellaris inferior
20 Tractus solitarius
21 Tractus spinalis nervi trigemini
22 Nervus accessorius, radices craniales
23 Fasciculus anterolateralis
24 Fibrae arcuatae internae
25 Fasciculus longitudinalis medialis
26 Decussation of fibrae arcuatae internae
27 Lemniscus medialis
28 Nervus hypoglossus
29 Amiculum olivae
30 Fibrae arcuatae externae
31 Tractus pyramidalis

Fig. 76. Section through the dorsal column nuclei (7/1 ×)

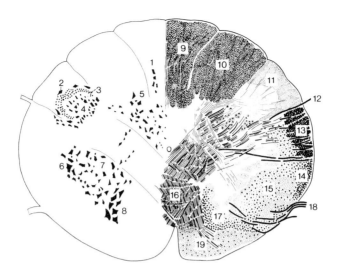

1 Nucleus gracilis
2 Cellulae marginales ⎫ Nucleus spinalis
3 Substantia gelatinosa ⎬ nervi trigemini,
4 Nucleus proprius ⎭ pars caudalis
5 Nucleus cuneatus medialis
6 Nucleus retroambiguus
7 Nucleus medullae oblongatae centralis
8 Nucleus supraspinalis

9 Fasciculus gracilis
10 Fasciculus cuneatus
11 Tractus spinalis nervi trigemini
12 Nervus accessorius, radices craniales
13 Tractus spinocerebellaris posterior
14 Tractus spinocerebellaris anterior
15 Fasciculus anterolateralis
16 Decussatio pyramidum
17 Fasciculus longitudinalis medialis
18 Nervus spinalis cervicalis I, radix ventralis
19 Tractus pyramidalis

Fig. 77. Section through the pyramidal decussation (7/1 ×)

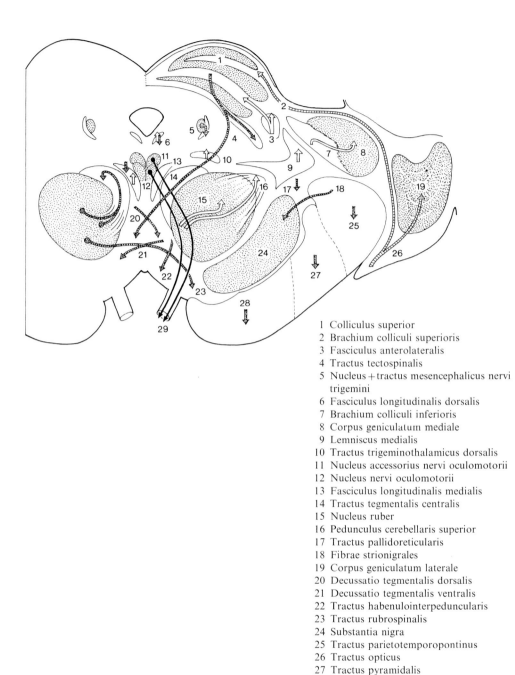

1 Colliculus superior
2 Brachium colliculi superioris
3 Fasciculus anterolateralis
4 Tractus tectospinalis
5 Nucleus + tractus mesencephalicus nervi
  trigemini
6 Fasciculus longitudinalis dorsalis
7 Brachium colliculi inferioris
8 Corpus geniculatum mediale
9 Lemniscus medialis
10 Tractus trigeminothalamicus dorsalis
11 Nucleus accessorius nervi oculomotorii
12 Nucleus nervi oculomotorii
13 Fasciculus longitudinalis medialis
14 Tractus tegmentalis centralis
15 Nucleus ruber
16 Pedunculus cerebellaris superior
17 Tractus pallidoreticularis
18 Fibrae strionigrales
19 Corpus geniculatum laterale
20 Decussatio tegmentalis dorsalis
21 Decussatio tegmentalis ventralis
22 Tractus habenulointerpeduncularis
23 Tractus rubrospinalis
24 Substantia nigra
25 Tractus parietotemporopontinus
26 Tractus opticus
27 Tractus pyramidalis
28 Tractus frontopontinus
29 Nervus oculomotorius

Fig. 78. Diagrammatic section through the superior colliculus, showing the course and direction of fibre tracts. Explanatory diagram to Figures 65–67

========== ascending tracts   ⬝⬝⬝⬝⬝⬝⬝⬝ sensory tracts
⬛⬛⬛⬛⬛⬛ descending tracts   ———— motor tracts

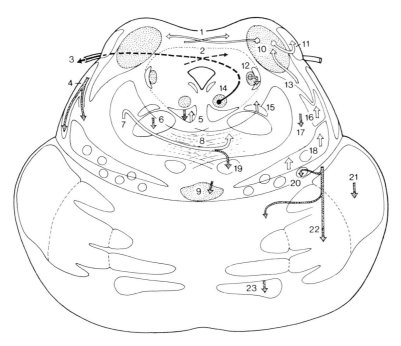

Fig. 79. Diagrammatic section through the inferior colliculus, showing the course and direction of fibre tracts. Explanatory diagram to Figure 69. Symbols as in Figure 78

1 Commissura colliculi inferioris
2 Decussatio nervorum trochlearium
3 Nervus trochlearis
4 Tractus tectopontinus
5 Fasciculus longitudinalis medialis
6 Tractus tegmentalis centralis
7 Pedunculus cerebellaris superior
8 Decussatio pedunculorum cerebellarium superiorum
9 Nucleus interpeduncularis

10 Colliculus inferior
11 Brachium colliculi inferioris
12 Nucleus + tractus mesencephalicus nervi trigemini
13 Lemniscus lateralis
14 Nucleus nervi trochlearis
15 Tractus trigeminothalamicus dorsalis
16 Fasciculus anterolateralis
17 Tractus pallidoreticularis
18 Lemniscus medialis
19 Pedunculus cerebellaris superior, ramus descendens
20 Fibrae corticotegmentales
21 Tractus parietotemporopontinus
22 Tractus pyramidalis
23 Tractus frontopontinus

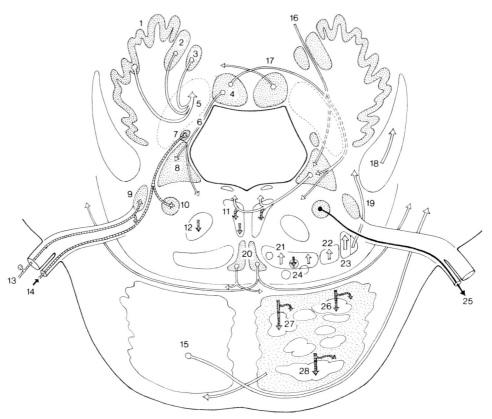

1 Nucleus dentatus
2 Nucleus emboliformis
3 Nucleus globosus
4 Nucleus fastigii
5 Pedunculus cerebellaris superior
6 Tractus fastigiobulbaris
7 Nucleus mesencephalicus nervi trigemini
8 Nuclei vestibulares
9 Nucleus sensorius principalis nervi trigemini
10 Nucleus motorius nervi trigemini
11 Fasciculus longitudinalis medialis
12 Tractus tegmentalis centralis
13 Radix sensoria nervi trigemini
14 Radix motoria nervi trigemini
   (fibrae proprioceptivae)
15 Nuclei pontis

16 Tractus corticovestibularis
17 Fasciculus uncinatus cerebelli
18 Pedunculus cerebellaris inferior
19 Tractus spinocerebellaris anterior
20 Nucleus reticularis tegmenti pontis +
   nucleus raphes pontis
21 Lemniscus medialis
22 Lemniscus lateralis
23 Fasciculus anterolateralis
24 Tractus corticobulbaris
25 Radix motoria nervi trigemini, fibrae
   motoriae
26 Tractus parietotemporopontinus
27 Tractus frontopontinus
28 Tractus pyramidalis

Fig. 80. Diagrammatic section through the cerebellar peduncles, showing the course and direction of fibre tracts. Explanatory diagram to Figure 71. Symbols as in Figure 78

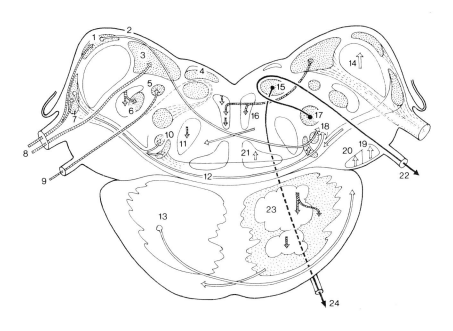

1 Nucleus cochlearis dorsalis
2 Striae acusticae dorsales
3 Nuclei vestibulares
4 Nucleus praepositus hypoglossi
5 Nucleus solitarius
6 Tractus + nucleus spinalis nervi trigemini
7 Nucleus cochlearis ventralis
8 Nervus vestibulocochlearis
9 Nervus intermedius
10 Oliva superior
11 Tractus tegmentalis centralis
12 Corpus trapezoideum
13 Nuclei pontis

14 Pedunculus cerebellaris inferior
15 Nucleus nervi abducentis
16 Fasciculus longitudinalis medialis
17 Nucleus nervi facialis
18 Lemniscus lateralis
19 Tractus spinocerebellaris anterior
20 Fasciculus anterolateralis
21 Lemniscus medialis
22 Nervus facialis
23 Tractus pyramidalis
24 Nervus abducens

Fig. 81. Diagrammatic section through cochlear nuclei and the trapezoid body, showing the course and direction of fibre tracts. Explanatory diagram to Figures 72–74. Symbols as in Figure 78

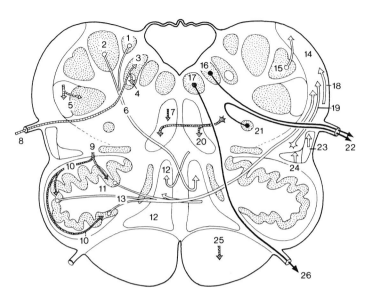

Fig. 82. Diagrammatic section through the medulla oblongata, showing the course and direction of fibre tracts. Explanatory diagram to Figures 75 and 76. Symbols as in Figure 78

1 Nucleus gracilis
2 Nucleus cuneatus medialis
3 Nucleus solitarius
4 Tractus solitarius
5 Tractus + nucleus spinalis nervi trigemini
6 Fibrae arcuatae internae
7 Fasciculus longitudinalis medialis
8 Nervus vagus, fibrae sensoriae
9 Tractus tegmentalis centralis
10 Amiculum olivae
11 Nucleus olivaris inferior
12 Lemniscus medialis
13 Tractus olivocerebellaris

14 Pedunculus cerebellaris inferior
15 Nucleus cuneatus lateralis
16 Nucleus dorsalis nervi vagi
17 Nucleus nervi hypoglossi
18 Tractus spinocerebellaris posterior
19 Tractus reticulocerebellaris
20 Tractus reticulospinalis
21 Nucleus ambiguus
22 Nervus vagus, fibrae motoriae
23 Tractus spinocerebellaris anterior
24 Fasciculus anterolateralis
25 Tractus pyramidalis
26 Nervus hypoglossus

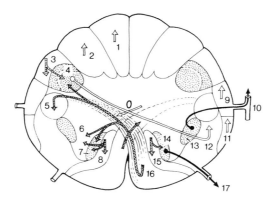

1 Fasciculus gracilis
2 Fasciculus cuneatus
3 Tractus spinalis nervi trigemini
4 Nucleus spinalis nervi trigemini
5 Tractus pyramidalis lateralis
6 Formatio reticularis
7 Nucleus supraspinalis
8 Fasciculus longitudinalis medialis

 9 Tractus spinocerebellaris posterior
10 Radix spinalis nervi accessorii
11 Tractus spinocerebellaris anterior
12 Fasciculus anterolateralis
13 Nucleus retroambiguus
14 Nucleus supraspinalis
15 Fasciculus longitudinalis medialis
16 Tractus pyramidalis
17 Radix ventralis nervi spinalis cervicalis I

Fig. 83. Diagrammatic section through the pyramidal decussation, showing the course and direction of fibre tracts. Explanatory diagram to Figure 77. Symbols as in Figure 78

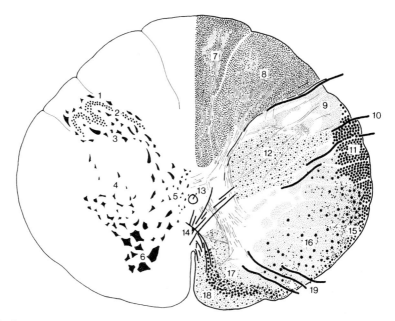

1 Cellulae marginales	7 Fasciculus gracilis
2 Substantia gelatinosa	8 Fasciculus cuneatus
3 Nucleus proprius	9 Fasciculus dorsolateralis
4 Processus reticularis	10 Radix spinalis nervi accessorii
5 Substantia intermedia	11 Tractus spinocerebellaris posterior
6 Cellulae motoriae	12 Tractus pyramidalis lateralis
	13 Canalis centralis
	14 Commissura alba
	15 Tractus spinocerebellaris anterior
	16 Fasciculus anterolateralis
	17 Fasciculus longitudinalis medialis
	18 Tractus pyramidalis anterior
	19 Radix ventralis

Fig. 84. Section through the first cervical segment (9/1 ×)

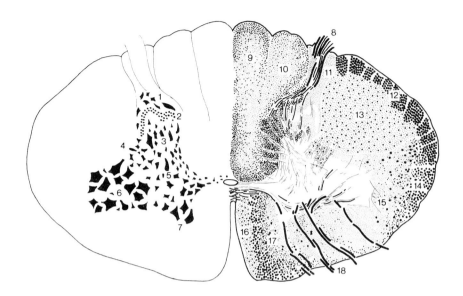

Fig. 85. Section through the transition of fifth to sixth cervical segment (9/1 ×)

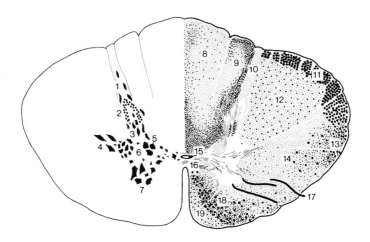

1 Cellulae marginales
2 Substantia gelatinosa
3 Nucleus proprius
4 Nucleus intermediolateralis
5 Nucleus thoracicus
6 Substantia intermedia
7 Cellulae motoriae

 8 Fasciculus gracilis
 9 Fasciculus cuneatus
10 Fasciculus dorsolateralis
11 Tractus spinocerebellaris posterior
12 Tractus pyramidalis lateralis
13 Tractus spinocerebellaris anterior
14 Fasciculus anterolateralis
15 Canalis centralis
16 Commissura alba
17 Radix ventralis
18 Fasciculus longitudinalis medialis
19 Tractus pyramidalis anterior

Fig. 86. Section through the fifth thoracic segment (9/1 ×)

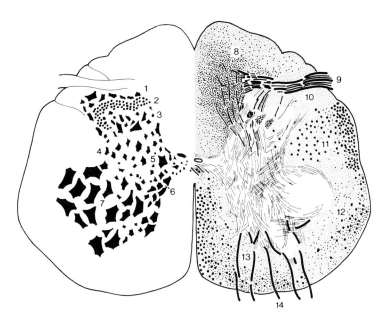

1 Cellulae marginales
2 Substantia gelatinosa
3 Nucleus proprius
4 Processus reticularis
5 Substantia intermedia
6 Nucleus cornucommissuralis
7 Cellulae motoriae laterales

8 Funiculus posterior
9 Radix dorsalis
10 Fasciculus dorsolateralis
11 Funiculus posterolateralis
12 Funiculus anterolateralis
13 Funiculus anterior
14 Radix ventralis

Fig. 87. Section through the fifth lumbar segment (9/1 ×)

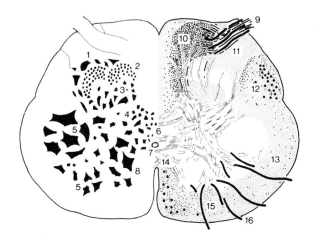

1 Cellulae marginales
2 Substantia gelatinosa
3 Nucleus proprius
4 Substantia intermedia
5 Cellulae motoriae laterales
6 Commissura grisea posterior
7 Commissura grisea anterior
8 Cellulae motoriae mediales

 9 Radix dorsalis
10 Funiculus posterior
11 Fasciculus dorsolateralis
12 Funiculus posterolateralis
13 Funiculus anterolateralis
14 Commissura alba
15 Funiculus anterior
16 Radix ventralis

Fig. 88. Section through the transition of fourth to fifth sacral segment (9/1 ×)

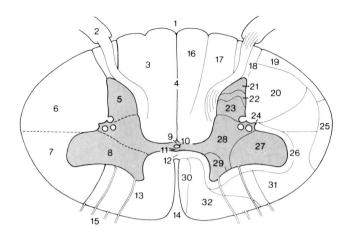

1 Sulcus medianus posterior
2 Radix dorsalis
3 Funiculus posterior
4 Septum medianum posterius
5 Cornu posterius
6 Funiculus posterolateralis ⎱ Funiculus
7 Funiculus anterolateralis ⎰ lateralis
8 Cornu anterius
9 Commissura grisea posterior
10 Canalis centralis
11 Commissura grisea anterior
12 Commissura alba
13 Funiculus anterior
14 Fissura mediana anterior
15 Radix ventralis

16 Fasciculus gracilis
17 Fasciculus cuneatus
18 Fasciculus dorsolateralis
19 Tractus spinocerebellaris posterior
20 Tractus pyramidalis lateralis
21 Cellulae marginales
22 Substantia gelatinosa
23 Nucleus proprius
24 Processus reticularis
25 Tractus spinocerebellaris anterior
26 Fasciculi proprii
27 Cellulae motoriae laterales
28 Substantia intermedia
29 Cellulae motoriae mediales
30 Tractus pyramidalis anterior
31 Fasciculus anterolateralis:
   Tractus spinoreticularis
   Tractus spinotectalis
   Tractus spinothalamicus
   Tractus spinoanularis
   Tractus spino-olivaris
32 Fasciculus longitudinalis medialis:
   Tractus vestibulospinalis medialis
   Tractus vestibulospinalis lateralis
   Tractus reticulospinalis
   Tractus tectospinalis
   Tractus interstitiospinalis

Fig. 89. The subdivision of the white and grey matter in the spinal cord

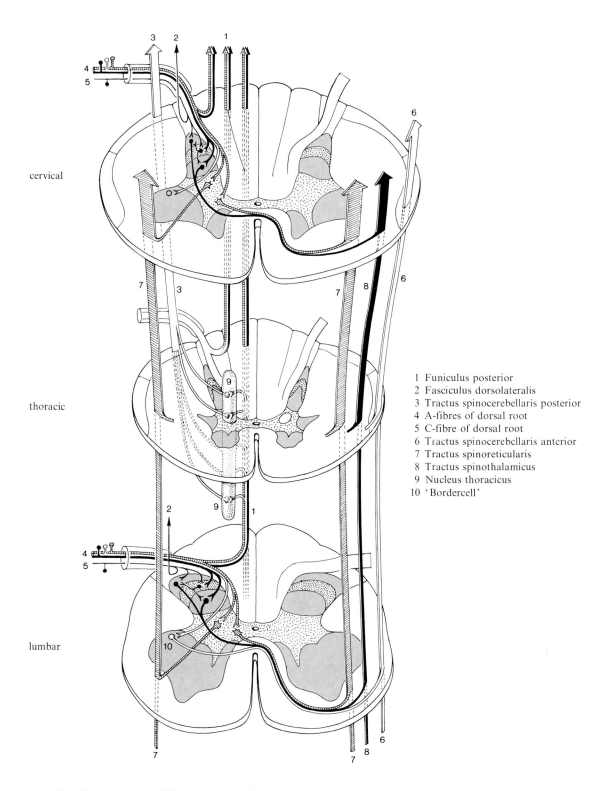

cervical

thoracic

lumbar

1 Funiculus posterior
2 Fasciculus dorsolateralis
3 Tractus spinocerebellaris posterior
4 A-fibres of dorsal root
5 C-fibre of dorsal root
6 Tractus spinocerebellaris anterior
7 Tractus spinoreticularis
8 Tractus spinothalamicus
9 Nucleus thoracicus
10 'Bordercell'

Fig. 90. The origin and localisation of the ascending fibre tracts at three levels of the spinal cord

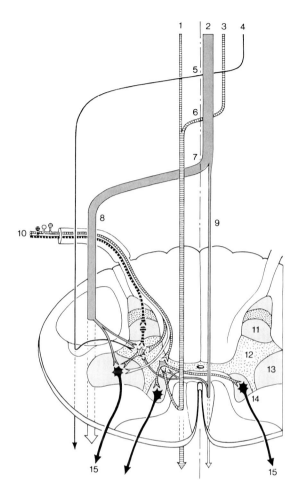

1 Fasciculus longitudinalis
  medialis dexter
2 Tractus pyramidalis
3 Fasciculus longitudinalis
  medialis sinister
4 Tractus rubrospinalis
5 Decussatio tegmentalis ventralis
  (mesencephali)
6 Decussatio tegmentalis
  metencephali
7 Decussatio pyramidum
8 Tractus pyramidalis lateralis
9 Tractus pyramidalis anterior
10 A-fibres of dorsal root
11 Nucleus proprius
12 Substantia intermedia
13 Cellulae motoriae laterales
14 Cellulae motoriae mediales
15 Radix ventralis

Fig. 91. Somatic reflex paths and descending supraspinal paths in the spinal cord; cervical level

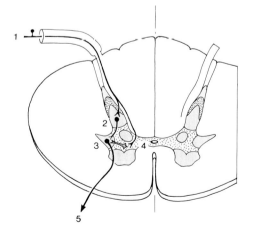

1 Visceral afferent fibre
2 Nucleus proprius
3 Nucleus intermediolateralis
4 Substantia intermedia
5 Visceral efferent fibre

Fig. 92. Visceral reflex paths in the spinal cord. Thoracic level

Part IV Functional Systems

Cranial Nerve Nuclei in the Brain Stem

The truncus cerebri or brain stem harbours the centres of origin and termination of ten (III–XII) of the twelve cranial nerves (Fig. 93). At first sight the arrangement of these cranial nerve nuclei does not show a definite pattern; however, the classical investigations of GASKELL [76, 77], HERRICK [96] and many others (for a review, see NIEUWENHUYS [186]) have revealed that these centres form part of functional zones, each of which is specifically related to one of the fibre categories of which the cranial nerves are composed. Before elucidating this zonal pattern the fibre categories or nerve components of peripheral nerves in general deserve some comment.

A single nerve fibre in a spinal or cranial nerve may be afferent or efferent and be concerned with the innervation of either somatic or visceral structures. Combination of these two subdivisions yields the following four categories of peripheral nerve fibres:

1) general somatic afferent fibres, which transmit impulses from the skin, skeletal muscles, joints and ligaments;

2) general visceral afferent fibres, which convey impulses from receptors in visceral organs and blood vessels centrally;

3) general visceral efferent fibres, which supply the smooth musculature of internal organs, the cardiac muscle and glands, and

4) general somatic efferent fibres, which innervate skeletal muscles derived from myotomes.

The denotation 'general' has been added because fibres belonging to these four categories occur in both spinal and cranial nerves. The cranial nerves may contain in addition nerve fibres related to special structures that occur in the head region. These fibres can be classed in the following three additional categories:

5) special somatic afferent fibres, which are associated with the receptors in the retina and in the cochlea;

6) special visceral afferent fibres, which supply the visceral sense organs, i.e., the organs of taste and smell, and

7) special visceral efferent fibres, which innervate muscles derived from the mesenchyme of the visceral, branchial arches.

Whereas a spinal nerve usually contains fibres of all four of the 'general' categories, there are wide variations between the cranial nerves as regards the types of fibres which they carry. Some of them have fibres of only one type, but in others fibres of two or more categories are present.

Returning now to the brain stem, the organisational pattern discovered by GASKELL and HERRICK and their followers is that the cranial nerve nuclei are essentially arranged in seven longitudinal zones and that each of these columns is specifically related to fibres of one of the categories mentioned above. Thus, as a cranial nerve composed of fibres of more than one type enters the brain, the fibres of its constituent types sort themselves out and pass to 'their own' specific zone.

The zonal or columnar pattern displayed by the cranial nerve nuclei in the brain stem is diagrammatically represented in Figure 94. As in the spinal cord, the afferent centres are situated in the alar lamina, whereas the efferent centres are located in the basal lamina. The sulcus limitans, which in the embryonic neuraxis marks the boundary between these two fundamental subdivisions, is in the adult only recognisable over a short extent. It will be noted that most of the zones are only partly occupied by cranial nerve nuclei. This may be related to the reduction of some components of some nerves during foetal development. The various zones and their constituent primary afferent or efferent centres will now be briefly reviewed, passing from lateral to medial.

The special somatic afferent (SSA) zone contains the nuclei of termination of the cochlear and vestibular division of the eighth nerve.

The general somatic afferent (GSA) zone includes the three sensory nuclei of the trigeminal nerve, i.e., the mesencephalic, the princeps or chief and the spinal nuclei. The latter nucleus, which also receives some fibres from the seventh, ninth and tenth nerves, is caudally continuous with the apical part of the dorsal horn of the spinal cord. The sensory trigeminal nuclei have shifted ventrolaterally during development, hence the princeps nucleus and the rostral part of the spinal nucleus lie in the adult ventral rather than medial to the vestibular nuclei.

The special visceral afferent (SVA) and general visceral afferent (GVA) zones are in the adult brain represented by a single cell mass, which receives the corresponding components of the seventh, ninth and tenth nerve. The latter unite in a well-defined fibre system, the tractus solitarius.

The general visceral efferent (GVE) zone contains four nuclei, the nucleus dorsalis of the tenth nerve, the nucleus salivatorius inferior and superior of the ninth and seventh nerve, respectively, and the accessory nucleus of the third nerve. These nuclei represent together the cranial division of the parasympathetic system. They give rise to preganglionic fibres that terminate in various autonomic ganglia.

The special visceral efferent (SVE) or branchiomotor zone contains the motor nuclei of the fifth and seventh nerve as well as the nucleus ambiguus, which gives rise to fibres that pass peripherally as components of the ninth, the tenth and the eleventh (cranial root) nerves. The spinal nucleus of the eleventh nerve, which is situated in the lateral part of the base of the ventral horn of the upper four cervical segments, also belongs to this zone. As with the general somatic afferent nuclei, the cell masses of the branchiomotor zone have migrated away from their original periventricular position.

The general somatic efferent (GSE) zone, finally, may be considered a rostral continuation of the anterior horn of the spinal cord. It comprises the nuclei of origin of the twelfth, sixth, fourth and third nerves. All four of these nuclei are located near the median plane of the brain stem.

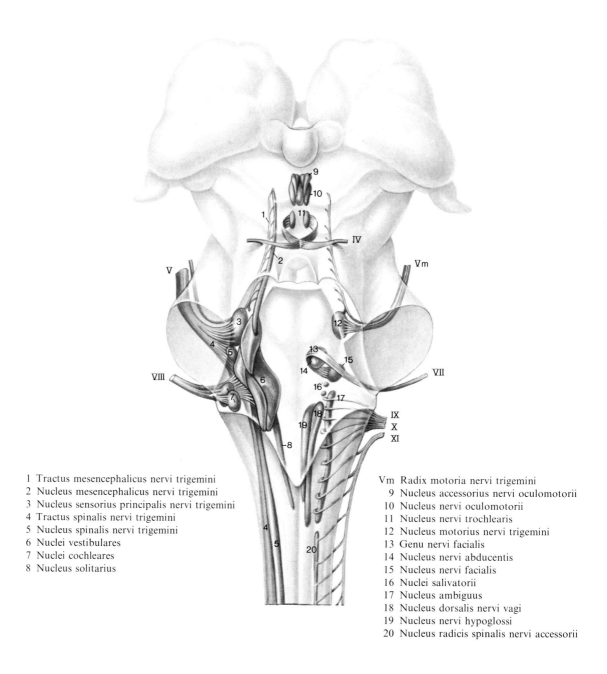

1 Tractus mesencephalicus nervi trigemini
2 Nucleus mesencephalicus nervi trigemini
3 Nucleus sensorius principalis nervi trigemini
4 Tractus spinalis nervi trigemini
5 Nucleus spinalis nervi trigemini
6 Nuclei vestibulares
7 Nuclei cochleares
8 Nucleus solitarius

Vm Radix motoria nervi trigemini
 9 Nucleus accessorius nervi oculomotorii
10 Nucleus nervi oculomotorii
11 Nucleus nervi trochlearis
12 Nucleus motorius nervi trigemini
13 Genu nervi facialis
14 Nucleus nervi abducentis
15 Nucleus nervi facialis
16 Nuclei salivatorii
17 Nucleus ambiguus
18 Nucleus dorsalis nervi vagi
19 Nucleus nervi hypoglossi
20 Nucleus radicis spinalis nervi accessorii

Fig. 93. The cranial nerve nuclei as viewed from the dorsal side (5/3 ×). *Left* sensory nuclei; *right* motor nuclei. *Roman numerals* indicate the corresponding cranial nerves

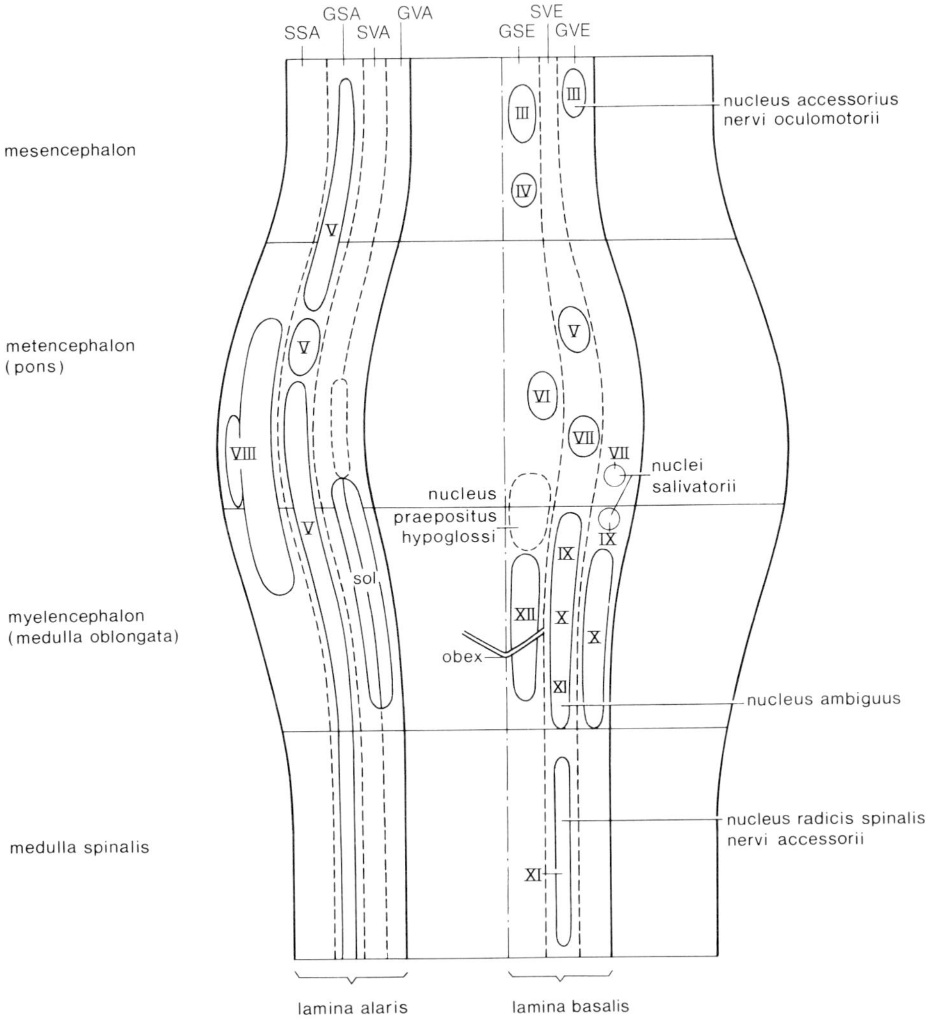

Fig. 94. Position of the cranial nerve nuclei in longitudinal columns. The *initials* at the *top* indicate the functional system to which each column belongs. The parts of the brain stem are indicated at *left*

General Sensory Systems and Taste

Sensory pathways within the central nervous system connect primary afferents with specific parts of the contralateral cerebral cortex. These so-called *lemniscal systems* synapse in nuclei in the spinal cord, the lower brain stem and in the sensory relay nuclei of the thalamus. Multisynaptic pathways through the reticular formation are arranged in parallel with the lemniscal systems. Reciprocal pathways from the cerebral cortex terminate in the main relay stations of the sensory projection systems. Protopathic systems, subserving pain and temperature and yielding ungraded, diffuse impressions of an all-or-none character, can be distinguished from epicritic systems concerned with the mediation of tactile and kinesthetic information of a discriminative type [31].

The Anterolateral System
(Figs. 95 and 96)

The *spinothalamic tract*, the protopathic pathway from the spinal cord, originates from marginal cells and cells of the nucleus proprius of the dorsal horn and from the intermediate grey [251]. *Spinoreticular fibres* arise from the same regions, but mainly from the intermediate grey matter [168]. Both myelinated A-fibres and unmyelinated C-fibres terminate on cells of the nucleus proprius and on cells of the substantia gelatinosa, which caps the dorsal horn. Marginal cells that are located in the dorsolateral fascicle outside the substantia gelatinosa receive exclusively C-fibres. A-fibres terminate both in the dorsal horn, in the intermediate grey and on the anterior horn cells. Axons of the substantia gelatinosa cells terminate on marginal cells and on the dendrites of the cells of the nucleus proprius. Together with C-fibres the axons of substantia gelatinosa cells constitute the dorsolateral fasciculus capping the dorsal horn [123, 146]. A-fibres ascend in the dorsal funiculus (cf. Fig. 90).

Spinothalamic fibres cross in the white commissure of the cord and ascend together with fibres of the spinoreticular and anterior spinocerebellar tracts in the anterolateral fasciculus. In the brain stem the anterolateral fasciculus is located lateral to the reticular formation. Spinoreticular fibres terminate at different levels in the medial reticular formation. They are the first link in a multisynaptic pathway that ascends within the reticular formation to terminate in the intralaminar nuclei of the thalamus. In addition, spinal fibres terminate in the central grey of the mesencephalon and in the magnocellular portion of the medial geniculate body. The spinothalamic tract terminates in the posterolateral ventral nucleus of the thalamus [124, 160, 163]. In their localisation in the anterolateral fasciculus and in their termination in the thalamus the ascending spinal fibres display a rough somatotopical organisation. Fibres from lower levels are located lateral to fibres originating from higher levels of the cord.

The Medial Lemniscus System
(Figs. 97 and 98)

The first link in the epicritic conduction pathway from the cord consists of ascending branches of dorsal root fibres in the posterior funiculus. In the posterior funiculus these fibres are somatotopically organised, fibres from sacral and lumbar roots ascend medially in the fasciculus gracilis, those from cervical roots laterally in the fasciculus cuneatus. A small contingent of thoracic fibres takes an intermediate position (Fig. 90). The gracile and cuneate fascicles terminate in corresponding nuclei in the caudal-most part of the medulla oblongata. From the gracile and the medial cuneate nuclei internal arcuate fibres originate which cross the midline and ascend in the medial lemniscus to terminate in the posterolateral ventral nucleus of the thalamus. This nucleus projects in a somatotopic manner to the sensory cortex in the postcentral gyrus.

The Trigeminal System
(Figs. 99 and 100)

Somatosensory fibres of the trigeminal nerve enter the pons in the sensory root (portio major) and are distributed over the principal sensory nucleus and the spinal trigeminal nucleus. A-fibres terminate in the principal sensory nucleus. A-fibres and C-fibres both descend in the spinal tract of the trigeminal nerve and terminate in its nucleus [57]. Small somatosensory components of the facial, glossopharyngeal and vagal nerves also join the spinal trigeminal tract. The pars caudalis of the spinal trigeminal nucleus consists of a substantia gelatinosa and a nucleus proprius and is continuous with the dorsal horn of the spinal grey matter. The synaptic relations of the A- and C-fibres of the spinal tract of the trigeminal nerve and those of the spinal roots are essentially similar.

The protopathic pathway from the trigeminal nerve, which joins the spinothalamic tract as the *lateral trigeminothalamic tract*, takes its origin from the pars caudalis of the spinal trigeminal nucleus and crosses in the caudal medulla oblongata [231]. The principal sensory nucleus gives rise to the crossed epicritic pathway, which joins the medial lemniscus as *trigeminal lemniscus* and the uncrossed, *dorsal trigeminothalamic tract* [233, 249]. The ascending trigeminothalamic connections terminate in the posteromedial -ventral nucleus of the thalamus, which projects to the ventral part of the postcentral gyrus.

Descending cortico-nuclear and cortico-spinal fibres from the postcentral gyrus terminate primarily contralaterally in the main sensory relay nuclei. This reciprocal connection is also somatotopically organised [139].

Contrary to all other primary afferents, the cells of origin of the proprioceptive, muscle spindle afferents, which enter the brain stem in the trigeminal nerve, are located within the central nervous system. They constitute the mesencephalic nucleus of the trigeminal nerve located alongside the central grey of the mesencephalon. The axons of these cells descend in the mesencephalic tract of the trigeminal nerve. Collaterals of the mesencephalic tract axons terminate on the cells of the motor nucleus of the trigeminal nerve. The main axons of the mesencephalic root, together with the axons of the motoneurons, constitute the motor root of the trigeminal nerve, which more distally joins the mandibular division of the trigeminal nerve.

The Visceral Afferent Systems
(Figs. 101 and 102)

Visceral afferent fibres and small contingents of somatosensory fibres enter the medulla oblongata in the facial, glossopharyngeal and vagal nerves. The somatosensory fibres join the spinal tract of the trigeminal nerve; more medially the visceral afferents descend in the solitary tract to terminate on the solitary nucleus. Special visceral afferents subserving taste terminate in the rostral, gustatory part of this nucleus. General visceral afferents descend farther caudally to terminate in the caudal, cardiorespiratory part of the solitary nucleus. Some of these fibres cross caudal to the obex and ascend over some distance in the contralateral solitary tract.

Ascending root fibres of the facial nerve terminate in the nucleus ovalis, a rostral prolongation of the solitary nucleus located dorsal to the sensory nuclei of the trigeminal nerve [214]. Fibres from the dorsal trigeminothalamic tract in man originate from the nucleus ovalis and the principal sensory nucleus of the trigeminal nerve. In the rat the ascending taste pathway contains an extra synapse in the medial parabrachial nucleus. From here fibres ascend bilaterally in the region of the dorsal trigeminothalamic tract to terminate in the medial parvocellular part of the posteromedial ventral nucleus of the thalamus [191, 192]. The cortical projection area for taste is found in the frontal and parietal operculum and in the limen insulae [18].

The dorsal longitudinal fascicle, located in the nucleus praepositus hypoglossi and the central grey, connects the caudal part of the solitary nucleus with the dorsal tegmental nucleus and more rostral structures [174]. Crossed, solitariospinal fibres descend from the caudal part of the nucleus [250].

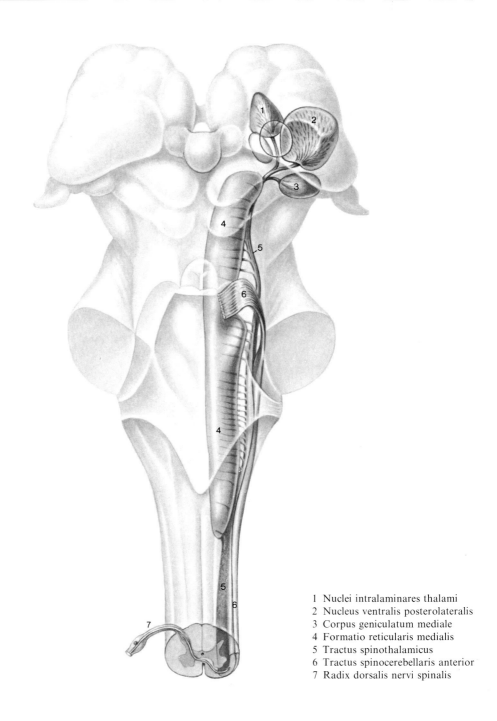

1 Nuclei intralaminares thalami
2 Nucleus ventralis posterolateralis
3 Corpus geniculatum mediale
4 Formatio reticularis medialis
5 Tractus spinothalamicus
6 Tractus spinocerebellaris anterior
7 Radix dorsalis nervi spinalis

Fig. 95. The anterolateral fasciculus. The position of the ascending spinal tracts and related nuclei in a dorsal view (5/3 ×)

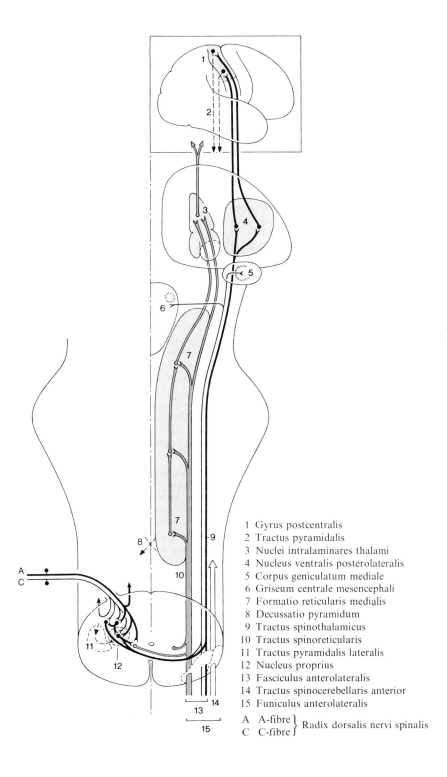

1 Gyrus postcentralis
2 Tractus pyramidalis
3 Nuclei intralaminares thalami
4 Nucleus ventralis posterolateralis
5 Corpus geniculatum mediale
6 Griseum centrale mesencephali
7 Formatio reticularis medialis
8 Decussatio pyramidum
9 Tractus spinothalamicus
10 Tractus spinoreticularis
11 Tractus pyramidalis lateralis
12 Nucleus proprius
13 Fasciculus anterolateralis
14 Tractus spinocerebellaris anterior
15 Funiculus anterolateralis

A A-fibre ⎱
C C-fibre ⎰ Radix dorsalis nervi spinalis

Fig. 96. The neuronal connections of the spinoreticular tract (*darkly shaded*) and of the spinothalamic tract (*solid line*)

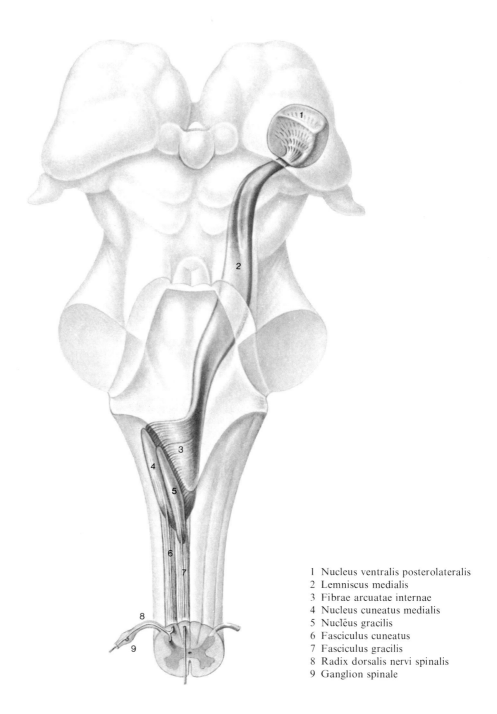

Fig. 97. The medial lemniscus. Position of tracts and nuclei in a dorsal view (5/3 ×)

1 Nucleus ventralis posterolateralis
2 Lemniscus medialis
3 Fibrae arcuatae internae
4 Nucleus cuneatus medialis
5 Nucleus gracilis
6 Fasciculus cuneatus
7 Fasciculus gracilis
8 Radix dorsalis nervi spinalis
9 Ganglion spinale

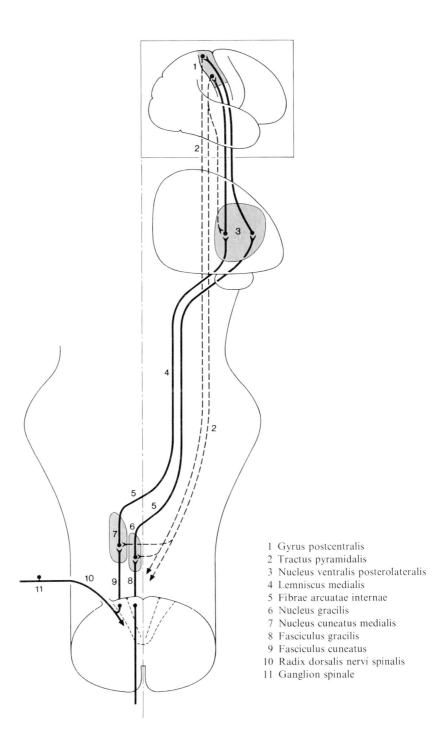

Fig. 98. The neuronal connections of the dorsal column nuclei and the medial lemniscus

1 Gyrus postcentralis
2 Tractus pyramidalis
3 Nucleus ventralis posterolateralis
4 Lemniscus medialis
5 Fibrae arcuatae internae
6 Nucleus gracilis
7 Nucleus cuneatus medialis
8 Fasciculus gracilis
9 Fasciculus cuneatus
10 Radix dorsalis nervi spinalis
11 Ganglion spinale

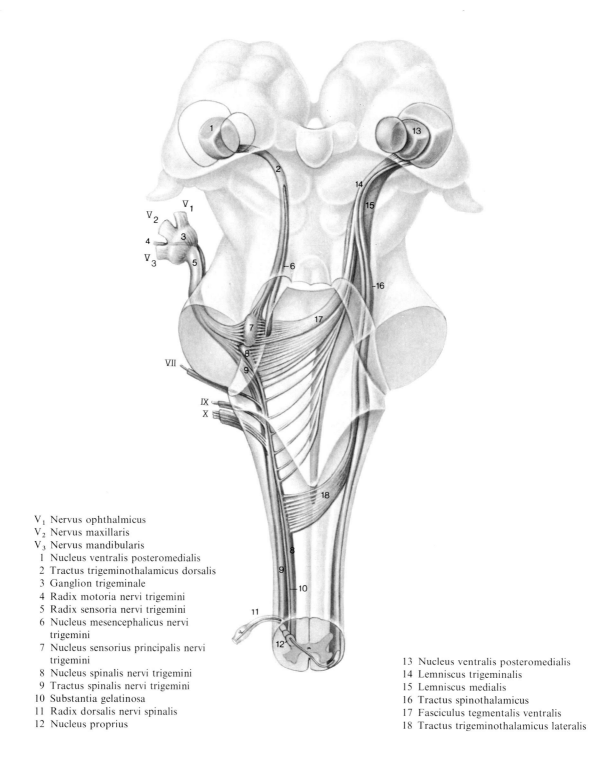

V₁ Nervus ophthalmicus
V₂ Nervus maxillaris
V₃ Nervus mandibularis
1 Nucleus ventralis posteromedialis
2 Tractus trigeminothalamicus dorsalis
3 Ganglion trigeminale
4 Radix motoria nervi trigemini
5 Radix sensoria nervi trigemini
6 Nucleus mesencephalicus nervi
  trigemini
7 Nucleus sensorius principalis nervi
  trigemini
8 Nucleus spinalis nervi trigemini
9 Tractus spinalis nervi trigemini
10 Substantia gelatinosa
11 Radix dorsalis nervi spinalis
12 Nucleus proprius

13 Nucleus ventralis posteromedialis
14 Lemniscus trigeminalis
15 Lemniscus medialis
16 Tractus spinothalamicus
17 Fasciculus tegmentalis ventralis
18 Tractus trigeminothalamicus lateralis

Fig. 99. The central connections of the trigeminal nerve. Position of nerves, tracts and nuclei in a dorsal view (5/3 ×). *Roman numerals* indicate the corresponding cranial nerves

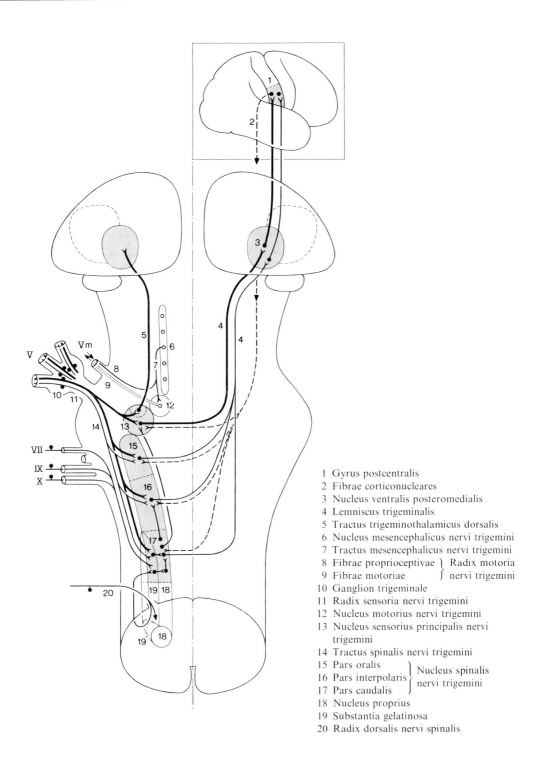

Fig. 100. The neuronal connections of the trigeminal nerve

1 Gyrus postcentralis
2 Fibrae corticonucleares
3 Nucleus ventralis posteromedialis
4 Lemniscus trigeminalis
5 Tractus trigeminothalamicus dorsalis
6 Nucleus mesencephalicus nervi trigemini
7 Tractus mesencephalicus nervi trigemini
8 Fibrae proprioceptivae ⎫ Radix motoria
9 Fibrae motoriae ⎭ nervi trigemini
10 Ganglion trigeminale
11 Radix sensoria nervi trigemini
12 Nucleus motorius nervi trigemini
13 Nucleus sensorius principalis nervi
    trigemini
14 Tractus spinalis nervi trigemini
15 Pars oralis ⎫ Nucleus spinalis
16 Pars interpolaris ⎬ nervi trigemini
17 Pars caudalis ⎭
18 Nucleus proprius
19 Substantia gelatinosa
20 Radix dorsalis nervi spinalis

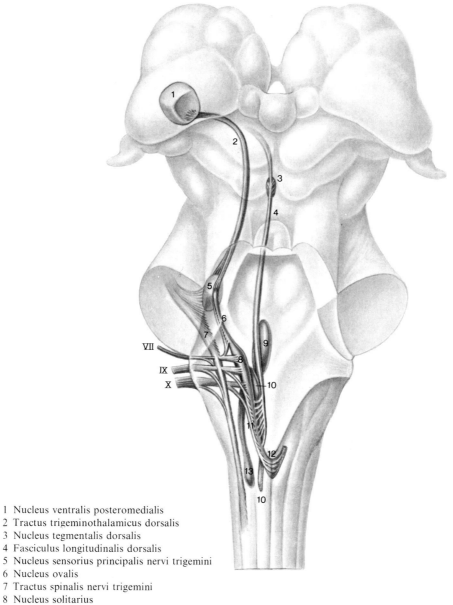

1 Nucleus ventralis posteromedialis
2 Tractus trigeminothalamicus dorsalis
3 Nucleus tegmentalis dorsalis
4 Fasciculus longitudinalis dorsalis
5 Nucleus sensorius principalis nervi trigemini
6 Nucleus ovalis
7 Tractus spinalis nervi trigemini
8 Nucleus solitarius
9 Nucleus praepositus hypoglossi
10 Nucleus dorsalis nervi vagi
11 Tractus solitarius
12 Obex
13 Nucleus ambiguus

Fig. 101. The tractus solitarius. Position of nerves, tracts and nuclei in a dorsal view (5/3 ×). *Roman numerals* indicate the corresponding cranial nerves

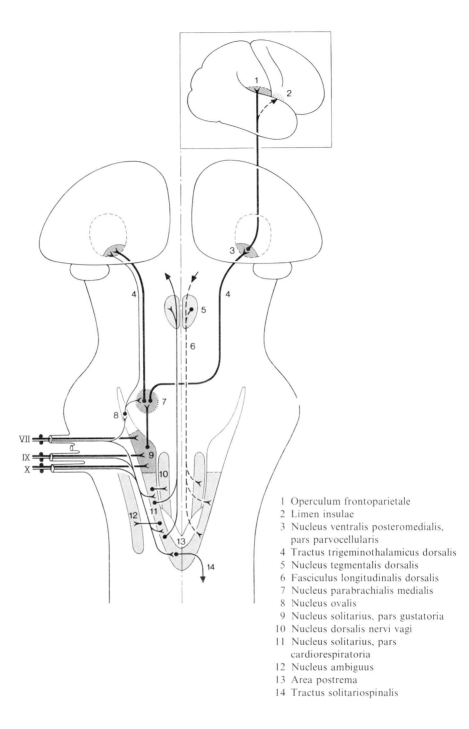

1 Operculum frontoparietale
2 Limen insulae
3 Nucleus ventralis posteromedialis,
   pars parvocellularis
4 Tractus trigeminothalamicus dorsalis
5 Nucleus tegmentalis dorsalis
6 Fasciculus longitudinalis dorsalis
7 Nucleus parabrachialis medialis
8 Nucleus ovalis
9 Nucleus solitarius, pars gustatoria
10 Nucleus dorsalis nervi vagi
11 Nucleus solitarius, pars
    cardiorespiratoria
12 Nucleus ambiguus
13 Area postrema
14 Tractus solitariospinalis

Fig. 102. The neuronal connections of the visceral afferent system. The nuclei of the special visceral afferent part of the system (taste) are *darkly shaded*

Special Sensory Systems

The Vestibular System

The first-order neurons in the vestibular system are bipolar neurons, the somata of which constitute the vestibular ganglion, located in the meatus acusticus internus. The peripheral processes of these elements are distributed to the hair cells of the cristae ampullares and of the maculae of the utriculus and sacculus. The central processes of these bipolar cells constitute the vestibular part of the VIIIth nerve, which enters the brain stem at the level of the junction of pons and medulla oblongata. Within the vestibular nuclear complex the fibres of the vestibular nerve diverge and form ascending and descending bundles. The nuclear complex mentioned comprises four cell masses, the superior, lateral, medial and inferior nuclei. The fibres of the ascending bundle of the vestibular nerve are peripherally related to the cristae ampullares. Centrally they terminate largely in the superior vestibular nucleus, but some ascend via the juxtarestiform body to the so-called vestibulocerebellum, i.e., the lobus flocculonodularis (Figs. 114 and 115). The fibres of the descending bundle of the vestibular nerve are distributed peripherally to the maculae sacculi and utriculi. Centrally these fibres constitute a conspicuous bundle in the nucleus inferior. Its fibres terminate in this nucleus and in the adjacent medial nucleus. The large-celled lateral vestibular nucleus or nucleus of Deiters receives only a few primary vestibular fibres in its central part. Contrary to the other vestibular nuclei it receives a large number of axons from Purkinje cells located in a paramedian strip of the cortex of the cerebellar vermis (Fig. 120). Because of this, the lateral vestibular nucleus may be considered a ventrally displaced cerebellar nucleus.

Apart from primary vestibular fibres the vestibular nuclei receive afferents from various other sources. Thus, the caudal parts of the medial and inferior nuclei receive a projection from the spinal cord and the same parts of these nuclei send fibres to the lobus flocculonodularis, thus forming a secondary vestibulocerebellar projection. Other afferents of the vestibular nuclei include (1) a strong input from the medial part of the cerebellar vermis, via bilateral pathways from the fastigial nuclei, and (2) fibres from the pontine and bulbar reticular formation [102] (Fig. 120).

As regards the efferent connections of the vestibular nuclei, the lateral vestibular nucleus gives rise to the lateral vestibulospinal tract, an ipsilateral, somatotopically organised bundle that descends in the lateral part of the anterior funiculus. Its fibres are distributed throughout the spinal cord, exerting facilitatory influences on spinal reflex activity and on extensor muscle tonus. The remaining three vestibular nuclei discharge efferents into the fasciculus longitudinalis medialis (f.l.m.), a conspicuous bundle extending in a dorsomedial position throughout the brain stem. Caudally this bundle passes over into the anterior funiculus of the spinal cord. Fibres originating from the medial and inferior vestibular nuclei constitute a descending component of the f.l.m. which is known as the medial vestibulospinal tract. By this connection, which does not extend beyond the midthoracic level, the muscles of the neck and upper extremities are brought under vestibular reflex control.

The ascending vestibular contributions to the f.l.m. originate mainly from the superior and medial nuclei. The fibres from the former remain on the ipsilateral side, whereas those from the latter ascend bilaterally. Together these fibres constitute the vestibulomesencephalic projection. They terminate in the nuclei of the extraocular muscles, i.e., the abducens, trochlear and oculomotor nuclei, and in the nucleus interstitialis of Cajal. The latter nucleus gives rise to a small interstitiospinal tract that, by way of the f.l.m. and the anterior funiculus, passes throughout the length of the brain stem and spinal cord. The fibres, connecting the vestibular nuclei with the oculomotor centres, are links in elementary three neuron reflex paths. The impulses conveyed by these paths help stabilise retinal images by producing eye movements compensatory for head movements.

The pathways along which vestibular stimuli reach the level of "conscious experience" are still imperfectly known. However, there is evidence that decussating secondary vestibular fibres, ascending beyond the f.l.m., terminate in the nucleus ventralis posterior inferior, a small but distinct thalamic nucleus, and that this cell mass gives rise to a thalamocortical projection. The latter presumably terminates in a small area buried in the anterior portion of the intraparietal sulcus [85, 73, 212].

Finally it should be mentioned that the vestibular nerve in addition to afferent fibres also carries some efferent fibres. The latter arise in some small cell groups, one of which is located in the lateral vestibular

nucleus and terminate in the vestibular organ. Presumably these efferent fibres exert an inhibitory influence on the transmission of vestibular impulses.

The Auditory System

The central auditory system includes in addition to several rhombencephalic cell masses a mesencephalic, a diencephalic and a telencephalic centre (Fig. 105). The rhombencephalic cell masses are the dorsal and ventral cochlear nuclei, the lateral and medial nuclei of the superior olivary complex, the nucleus of the corpus trapezoideum and the nucleus of the lemniscus lateralis. At the mesencephalic level the auditory system is represented by the inferior colliculus. The specific diencephalic nucleus for hearing is the medial geniculate body, which forms part of the dorsal thalamus. The telencephalic auditory centre is located in the temporal part of the neocortex, more specifically in the two transverse convolutions of Heschl, which form part of the floor of the lateral sulcus.

Figure 105 shows that the centres just mentioned are interconnected by distinct fibre streams. The cochlear nuclei give rise to two, more-or-less transversely orientated bundles, the corpus trapezoideum and the striae acusticae dorsales. The corpus trapezoideum crosses in the ventral part of the tegmentum. After having attained the lateral part of the pons, this bundle turns abruptly rostralward and continues as the lateral lemniscus. The nuclei of the superior olivary complex and the cell mass bearing its name lie embedded in the corpus trapezoideum. The striae acusticae dorsales pass over the inferior cerebellar peduncle. Arching ventrally, this bundle traverses the reticular formation to reach the region of the contralateral superior olivary complex where it passes over into the lateral lemniscus. The bundle just mentioned is situated in the dorsolateral part of the pons and the caudal midbrain. It ascends to the inferior colliculus, in which most of its fibres terminate. The brachium colliculi inferioris, a prominent bundle visible on the surface of the midbrain, connects the inferior colliculus with the medial geniculate body. The inferior colliculi of both sides are, in addition, interconnected by commissural fibres. The final link in the auditory system is formed by the auditory radiation through which the medial geniculate body is connected with the cerebral cortex. Passing laterally, this radiation traverses the sublenticular portion of the internal capsule.

The primary neurons of the auditory system are bipolar cells that together constitute the ganglion spirale. Their peripheral processes make contact with the bases of the outer and inner hair cells in the organ of Corti. The central processes of the bipolar cells constitute the cochlear division of the VIIIth nerve, which enters the central nervous system just caudal to the vestibular portion of the same nerve. The primary auditory fibres dichotomise immediately after their entrance into an ascending and a descending branch. The descending branches pass to the dorsal cochlear nucleus, situated dorsal to the inferior cerebellar peduncle, whereas the ascending branches enter the ventral cochlear nucleus, situated ventrolaterally to that peduncle.

Secondary auditory fibres originating from the dorsal cochlear nucleus constitute the striae acusticae dorsales and pass via this bundle and via the lateral lemniscus to the contralateral inferior colliculus.

The other secondary auditory projection, the corpus trapezoideum, arises from the ventral cochlear nucleus. A certain proportion of its fibres passes, like those of the dorsal auditory striae, directly to the inferior colliculus, but many other fibres are interrupted in one of the nuclei that lie embedded in this bundle or in the nucleus of the lateral lemniscus. Thus, the pathway from the ventral cochlear nucleus to the inferior colliculus has both direct and multisynaptic components (Fig. 106). It has recently been established [236] that in the chimpanzee some secondary auditory fibres pass uninterruptedly to the medial geniculate body. The neuronal links interconnecting the inferior colliculus, the medial geniculate body and the auditory cortex do not deserve further comment; it is, however, important to note that the auditory cortex receives not only impulses from the contralateral cochlea but also from the ipsilateral cochlea. The ipsilateral projection is provided by efferents from the ventral cochlear nucleus which, after a synaptic interruption in the ipsilateral superior olivary complex, pass to the ipsilateral lateral lemniscus. Fibres conveying impulses from the contralateral side back to the ipsilateral side, several of which are indicated in Figure 106, are probably also involved.

Parallel with the pathway from the organ of Corti to the auditory cortex, there is an uninterrupted chain of neurons conducting impulses in the opposite direction. The final link in this descending system is formed by the olivo-cochlear bundle of Rasmussen, which originates from some small cell groups situated in the vicinity of the superior olivary nuclei. Part of the fibres of this bundle decussate in the tegmentum. They enter the vestibular nerve and join the cochlear nerve via a vestibulocochlear anastomosis. After having entered the cochlea, they terminate at the bases of the hair cells in the organ of Corti. Physiological experiments have shown that these fibres exert an inhibitory influence on the sensory outflow from the cochlea.

The auditory cell masses in the brain stem serve not only as relay nuclei, but also as reflex centres. Thus, fibres passing from the medial superior olivary nucleus to the motor nuclei of the trigeminal and facial nerves form part of reflex paths that link the organ of Corti with the tensor tympani and the stapedius muscles. In response to sounds of high intensity, these muscles contract reflexly and dampen the vibration of the ear ossicles. In this way the organ of Corti is protected from damage by excessive stimulation. Fibres passing from the inferior colliculus to the superior colliculus are considered important links in the pathway providing for reflex turning of eyes and head in response to auditory stimuli (Fig. 111 C).

The Visual System

The Visual Pathway (Figs. 107 and 108)

The visual pathway begins at the retina, a thin, transparent lamina of tissue that ontogenetically is derived from the wall of the diencephalon. The retina is a laminated structure that contains photoreceptor cells, neurons and glia. The photoreceptors, i.e., the rods and cones, constitute the outer layer of the retina. Impulses from these elements are transmitted to bipolar cells that form an intermediate zone. These elements represent the primary afferent neurons of the visual system. Contrary to the corresponding elements in other sensory systems, the retinal bipolar cells are provided with only very short axons. These processes terminate on the ganglion cells, large elements that occupy the inner zone of the retina. The axons of the ganglion cells pass over the inner surface of the retina and converge towards the posterior pole of the eye, where they pierce through foramina in the sclera and then constitute the optic nerve. Only

after having left the retina the axons of the ganglion cells acquire a myelin sheath. The optic nerves pass to the optic chiasm, which is situated at the base of the brain in the most rostral part of the hypothalamus (Fig. 107). Within the optic chiasm a partial decussation takes place, fibres from the nasal halves of the retinae crossing to the opposite side and those from the temporal halves of the retinae remaining uncrossed. After this partial decussation the axons of the retinal ganglion cells continue without interruption behind the chiasma as two diverging optic tracts. These arch around the lateral sides of the diencephalon until they reach the lateral geniculate bodies, where most of their fibres terminate. However, a small number of fibres continue in a mediocaudal direction and pass via the brachium of the superior colliculus to the superior colliculus and to the pretectal area (Fig. 108). These fibres link the visual system with the centres that regulate the activity of the intrinsic and extrinsic musculature of the eye. Moreover, the retinotectal fibres form part of an alternative ("extrageniculate") projection to the cerebral cortex.

It is noteworthy that some retinofugal fibres or collaterals leave the optic pathway already at the level of the optic chiasm, to enter the anterior part of the hypothalamus. These fibres terminate in the suprachiasmatic nucleus, a small periventricular cell mass that, as its name implies, lies directly above the chiasm [45, 170, 246]. Via this retinohypothalamic projection the visual system participates in the regulation of various behavioural rhythms [170].

As has already been mentioned, most fibres of the optic tract end in the lateral geniculate body. This thalamic centre contains six layers of cells upon which the retinal fibres terminate in a highly orderly fashion, layers 2, 3 and 5 receiving fibres from the ipsilateral eye and layers 1, 4 and 6 from the contralateral eye.

The efferent fibres of the lateral geniculate body constitute the optic radiation or geniculocalcarine tract, which terminates in the primary visual area of the cerebral cortex. This area, which is known as the area striata, surrounds the calcarine sulcus on the medial side of the occipital lobe. The fibres of the optic radiation first traverse the retrolenticular part of the internal capsule then arch around the lateral ventricle and finally pass posteriorly towards the occipital cortex. Figure 107 shows that a large proportion of the fibres of the optic radiation do not reach their destination by the shortest route. Those arising from the lateral part of the lateral geniculate body sweep forward into the temporal lobe and pass laterally over the inferior horn of the lateral ventricle before turning backwards.

There is a precise point-to-point projection from the retina to the lateral geniculate body and from the latter to the visual cortex. Figure 108 illustrates some features of these projections in relation to the projection of the external world ('visual field') on the retina.

1. As a consequence of the partial decussation of the retinofugal fibres in the chiasm, all impulses from the right halves of both retinae (representing the left half of the visual field) are transmitted to the right occipital lobe and vice versa.

2. The lower retinal halves (representing the upper half of the visual field) project to the primary visual cortex inferior to the calcarine sulcus, while the upper halves of the retinae project to the cortex above that sulcus.

3. The maculae, i.e. the retinal areas concerned in central vision project to a relatively very large area, which forms the posterior part of the primary visual cortex.

The parts of the retinae corresponding to the peripheral part of the binocular field project to a smaller intermediate portion of the primary visual cortex, whereas the most peripheral nasal parts of the retinae that correspond to the most temporal parts of the visual field in which vision is monocular project to the extreme anterior part of the visual cortical area.

The primary visual cortex (area 17) projects to the surrounding secondary visual or visual association cortex (areae 18 and 19). The retino-geniculo-calcarine projection is parallelled by a second pathway that, because its fibres do not synapse in the lateral geniculate body, is designated as the extrageniculate visual pathway. The successive links in this pathway are (1) retinotectal fibres, (2) fibres, originating from the superficial layers of the colliculus superior, which project to certain parts of the pulvinar, and (3) fibres passing from this thalamic centre to both the primary and secondary visual cortical fields.

Visual Reflexes

The light reflex, i.e., constriction of the pupil on illumination of the eye, is mediated by a reflex arc that involves the following links (Fig. 109): (1) axons of retinal ganglion cells which pass via the optic nerve and tract to the pretectal area, (2) axons of pretectal neurons, projecting to the accessory oculomotor nuclei (nuclei of Edinger-Westphal) of the same and opposite side [17], (3) axons of the parasympathetic preganglionic neurons of the nuclei just mentioned, which pass with the oculomotor nerves to the ciliary ganglia where they synapse with (4) postganglionic neurons whose axons innervate the sphincter pupillae muscle of the iris. The pretectal efferents to the ipsilateral accessory oculomotor nucleus provide for the direct pupillary light reflex, those to the contralateral nucleus for the consensual pupillary light reflex.

In addition to the response to light, pupillary constriction also occurs following the initiation of ocular convergence. The neural pathway for this convergence-induced pupillary constriction is believed to be independent of that for light-induced pupillary constriction since the two reflexes can be observed to be dissociated in clinical cases (Argyll Robertson's sign).

The centre for pupillary dilatation is located in the intermediolateral cell column of the upper thoracic cord (Fig. 109). The preganglionic sympathetic fibres originating from this so-called ciliospinal centre ascend through the sympathetic trunk and synapse in the superior cervical ganglion with postganglionic elements. The axons of the latter pass along the branches of the internal carotid artery and traverse the ciliary ganglion before they innervate the dilatator pupillae muscle of the iris. Fibres descending through the lateral part of the medulla oblongata and of the spinal cord synapse on the cells of the sympathetic ciliospinal centre. The origin of these fibres is unknown.

The pathway for the accommodation reflex, i.e., increase of the curvature of the lens for near vision, so far as its mesencephalic centres and efferent limb are concerned, is closely comparable to the pathway for the light reflex. In both pathways the pretectal area, the accessory oculomotor nucleus and the ciliary ganglion are successive relay stations. However, the afferent limb of the accommodation reflex includes the visual cortex and is thus much longer and much more complex than that of the light reflex (Fig. 110). The final link on the efferent side of the accommodation pathway is formed by the postganglionic fibres to the ciliary muscle.

Eye Movements

Eye movements are effected by the coordinated activity of the six extraocular muscles. These muscles are innervated by the third, fourth and sixth cranial nerves, the nuclei of which are located in the medial part of the pontine and mesencephalic tegmentum. We still lack a coherent picture of the central neural mechanism for the control of the eye movements; however, the following features of the circuitry involved are well established.

1. The abducens and oculomotor nuclei contain, in addition to motor neurons, 'premotor' interneurons, which provide reciprocal internuclear pathways [13, 80, 81, 158] (Fig. 111A: *open circles*). The interneurons of the abducens nucleus synapse with the motoneurons within the same nucleus and project to the contralateral oculomotor complex, where they terminate on the motoneurons of the rectus medialis muscle. This "six-to-three pathway" is most probably responsible for mediating conjugate lateral gaze and thereby for the syndrome of anterior internuclear ophthalmoplegia [13].

2. Physiological and clinical evidence suggests that a group of cells located in the paramedian pontine reticular formation (PPRF) is intimately associated with the control of horizontal gaze movements [98]. It has been shown that this centre projects to the ipsilateral abducens and praepositus hypoglossi nuclei (Fig. 111A). This finding renders it likely that the PPRF centre exerts its control of horizontal gaze by means of these descending connections, rather than by direct impulse conduction to the oculomotor complex [80].

3. The vestibular nuclear complex sends a massive, bilateral projection to the nuclei of the extraocular muscles (Fig. 104). This projection is so organised that the ipsi-

lateral connections are inhibitory and the contralateral connections are excitatory [10, 13]. These connections form part of vestibulo-ocular reflex pathways. The impulses transmitted along these pathways help stabilise the visual world on the retina by producing eye movements compensatory for head movements.

4. The nucleus praepositus hypoglossi discharges fibres to all of the external eye muscle nuclei, both ipsilateral and contralateral, and has to be considered therefore an important 'preoculomotor' centre [11, 81, 157] (Fig. 111B). The praepositus nucleus receives afferents from the ipsilateral and contralateral vestibular complex, which, so far as excitation and inhibition are concerned, are similarly organised as the vestibulo-oculomotor projections [10]. Other connections of the praepositus nucleus include a projection from the ipsilateral interstitial nucleus of Cajal [39] and a reciprocal relation with the cerebellum [7, 128, 264]. Physiological experiments [12] indicate that the nucleus praepositus hypoglossi plays a significant role in the generation of rapid vertical and horizontal eye movements, as well as in fixation and vestibular or visually guided pursuit movements of the eyes.

5. The interstitial nucleus of Cajal also represents a preoculomotor centre (Fig. 111C). This nucleus receives afferents from the vestibular nuclei, from the pretectal area and from the superior colliculus [3, 135]. Cortical afferents emanating from area 8 (the 'frontal eye field') have also been described [9]. The efferents of the interstitial nucleus pass to the oculomotor and trochlear nuclei of both sides and, as mentioned above, to the ipsilateral nucleus praepositus hypoglossi [39].

6. The superior colliculus receives visual, auditory as well as somatosensory stimuli and is involved in the reflex turning of the head and eyes towards the source of these stimuli. The visual information originates in part directly from both eyes and in part from the ipsilateral visual cortex. The auditory and somatosensory stimuli reach the superior colliculus by way of projections originating from the inferior colliculus and the spinal cord, respectively (Fig. 111C). Efferents of the superior colliculus gain access to the external eye muscle nuclei via the interstitial nucleus and preoculomotor cells in the reticular formation. The projection to the latter cells forms part of the predorsal fascicle, a large decussating bundle that descends near the median raphe just ventral to the medial longitudinal fascicle.

7. The pretectal area is not only involved in the accommodative and pupillary reflexes, but is also implicated in the mechanism of oculomotor control. Clinical evidence suggests that the vertical eye movements have special representation in the pretectum. The efferent pathways involved include bilateral connections with the interstitial nucleus of Cajal and a widespread projection to the ipsilateral superior colliculus [135] (Fig. 111C).

Interestingly, the pretectal area also projects to the ipsilateral inferior olive. This connection probably provides a link in a pathway whereby visual information gains access to the vestibulocerebellum to influence cerebellar modulation of the vestibulo-ocular reflex [32, 110].

8. A small cortical area situated in the posterior part of the middle frontal gyrus is concerned with voluntary eye movements, not dependent on visual stimuli ('scanning'). The initial part of the pathway from this frontal cortical eye field (roughly: area 8) to the nuclei of the extraocular muscles is formed by fibres that terminate in the pretectal area and in the superior colliculus [135] (Fig. 111C).

9. A large occipital cortical field, roughly corresponding to areae 17, 18 and 19, plays a role in the control of movements of the eyes which are induced by visual stimuli ('pursuit movements'). This occipital eye field sends, just as the frontal eye field, efferents to the superior colliculus and to the pretectum [14, 255].

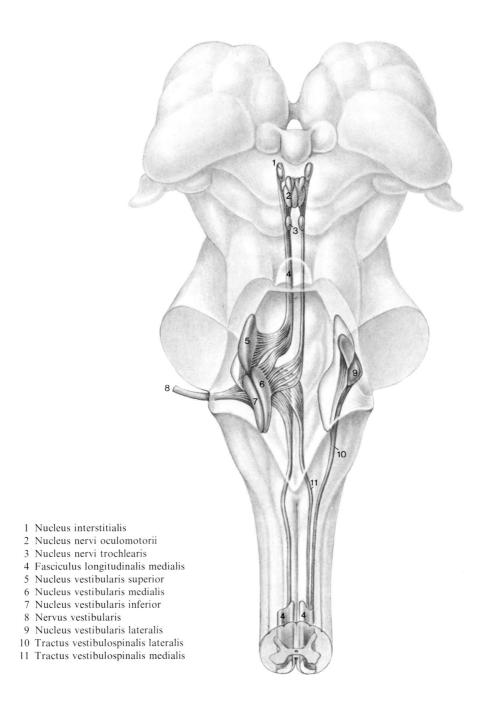

1 Nucleus interstitialis
2 Nucleus nervi oculomotorii
3 Nucleus nervi trochlearis
4 Fasciculus longitudinalis medialis
5 Nucleus vestibularis superior
6 Nucleus vestibularis medialis
7 Nucleus vestibularis inferior
8 Nervus vestibularis
9 Nucleus vestibularis lateralis
10 Tractus vestibulospinalis lateralis
11 Tractus vestibulospinalis medialis

Fig. 103. The vestibular system. Position of nerve, tracts and nuclei in a dorsal view (5/3 ×).
The lateral vestibulospinal tract is shown on the *right*

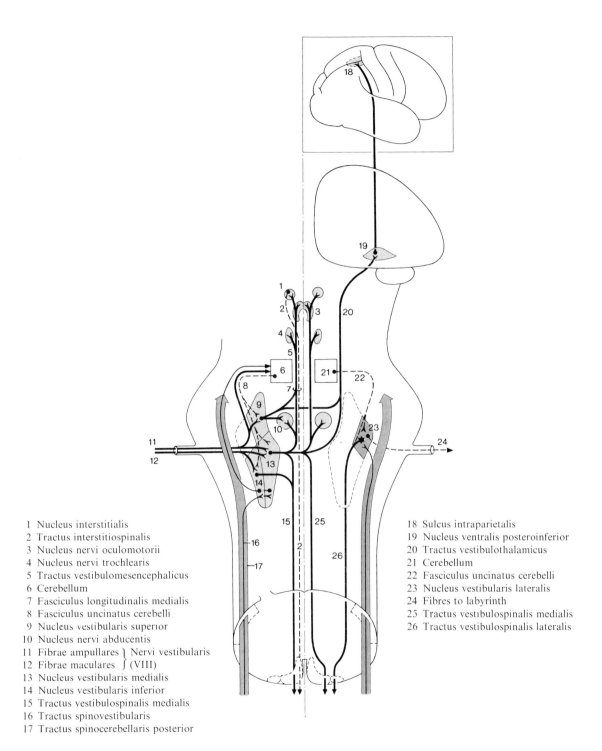

1 Nucleus interstitialis
2 Tractus interstitiospinalis
3 Nucleus nervi oculomotorii
4 Nucleus nervi trochlearis
5 Tractus vestibulomesencephalicus
6 Cerebellum
7 Fasciculus longitudinalis medialis
8 Fasciculus uncinatus cerebelli
9 Nucleus vestibularis superior
10 Nucleus nervi abducentis
11 Fibrae ampullares ⎫ Nervi vestibularis
12 Fibrae maculares ⎭ (VIII)
13 Nucleus vestibularis medialis
14 Nucleus vestibularis inferior
15 Tractus vestibulospinalis medialis
16 Tractus spinovestibularis
17 Tractus spinocerebellaris posterior

18 Sulcus intraparietalis
19 Nucleus ventralis posteroinferior
20 Tractus vestibulothalamicus
21 Cerebellum
22 Fasciculus uncinatus cerebelli
23 Nucleus vestibularis lateralis
24 Fibres to labyrinth
25 Tractus vestibulospinalis medialis
26 Tractus vestibulospinalis lateralis

Fig. 104. The neuronal connections of the vestibular system. For connections with the cerebellum see also Figures 115 and 120

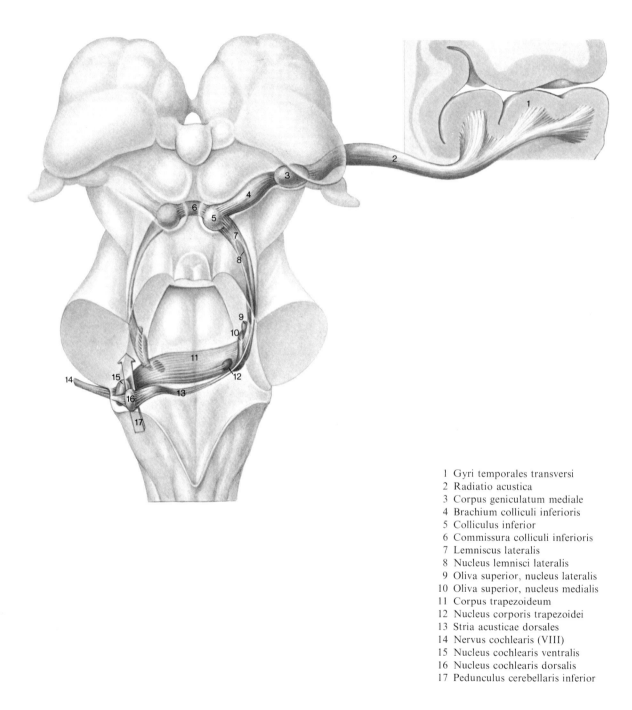

Fig. 105. The auditory system. Position of nerve, nuclei and tracts in a dorsal view (5/3 ×). The transverse temporal gyri of Heschl have been drawn in the true position relative to the brain stem and the thalamus

1 Gyri temporales transversi
2 Radiatio acustica
3 Corpus geniculatum mediale
4 Brachium colliculi inferioris
5 Colliculus inferior
6 Commissura colliculi inferioris
7 Lemniscus lateralis
8 Nucleus lemnisci lateralis
9 Oliva superior, nucleus lateralis
10 Oliva superior, nucleus medialis
11 Corpus trapezoideum
12 Nucleus corporis trapezoidei
13 Stria acusticae dorsales
14 Nervus cochlearis (VIII)
15 Nucleus cochlearis ventralis
16 Nucleus cochlearis dorsalis
17 Pedunculus cerebellaris inferior

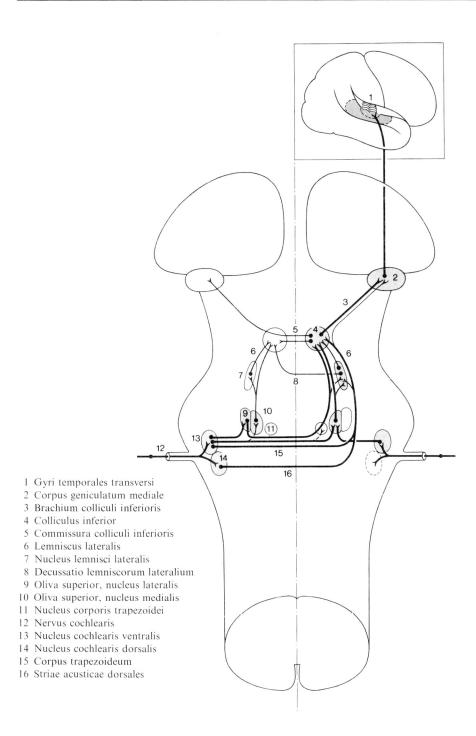

1 Gyri temporales transversi
2 Corpus geniculatum mediale
3 Brachium colliculi inferioris
4 Colliculus inferior
5 Commissura colliculi inferioris
6 Lemniscus lateralis
7 Nucleus lemnisci lateralis
8 Decussatio lemniscorum lateralium
9 Oliva superior, nucleus lateralis
10 Oliva superior, nucleus medialis
11 Nucleus corporis trapezoidei
12 Nervus cochlearis
13 Nucleus cochlearis ventralis
14 Nucleus cochlearis dorsalis
15 Corpus trapezoideum
16 Striae acusticae dorsales

Fig. 106. The neuronal connections of the auditory system

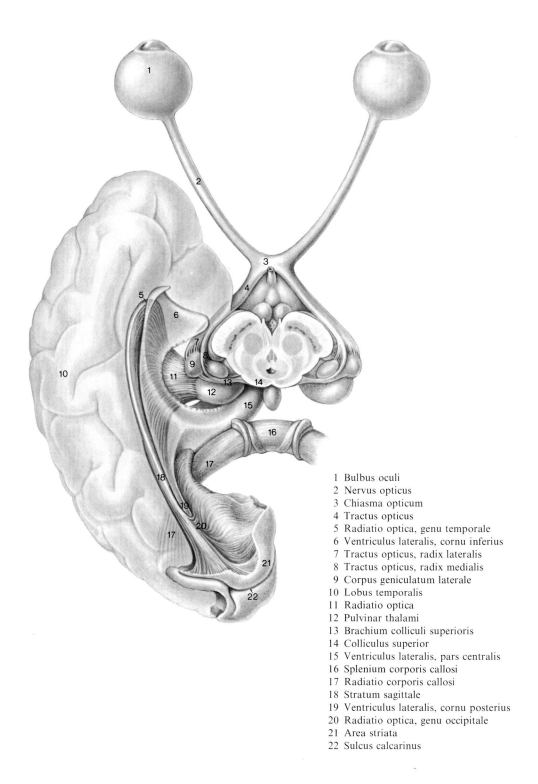

1 Bulbus oculi
2 Nervus opticus
3 Chiasma opticum
4 Tractus opticus
5 Radiatio optica, genu temporale
6 Ventriculus lateralis, cornu inferius
7 Tractus opticus, radix lateralis
8 Tractus opticus, radix medialis
9 Corpus geniculatum laterale
10 Lobus temporalis
11 Radiatio optica
12 Pulvinar thalami
13 Brachium colliculi superioris
14 Colliculus superior
15 Ventriculus lateralis, pars centralis
16 Splenium corporis callosi
17 Radiatio corporis callosi
18 Stratum sagittale
19 Ventriculus lateralis, cornu posterius
20 Radiatio optica, genu occipitale
21 Area striata
22 Sulcus calcarinus

Fig. 107. The visual system I: the retinogeniculocortical projection in a ventral view (1/1 ×). Of the cerebral hemispheres only the right temporal lobe has been depicted

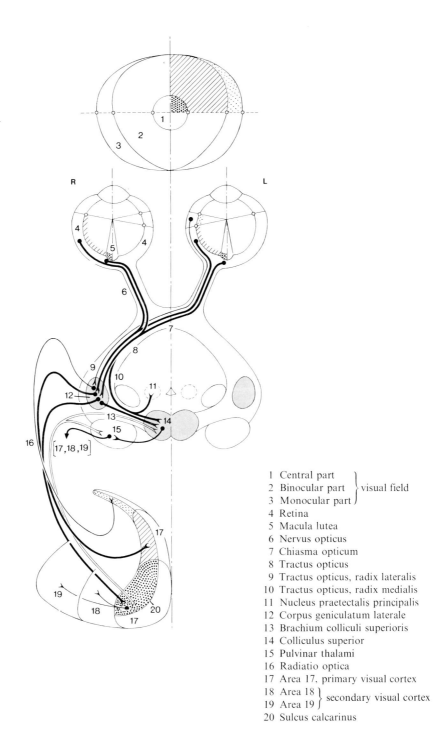

1	Central part
2	Binocular part } visual field
3	Monocular part
4	Retina
5	Macula lutea
6	Nervus opticus
7	Chiasma opticum
8	Tractus opticus
9	Tractus opticus, radix lateralis
10	Tractus opticus, radix medialis
11	Nucleus praetectalis principalis
12	Corpus geniculatum laterale
13	Brachium colliculi superioris
14	Colliculus superior
15	Pulvinar thalami
16	Radiatio optica
17	Area 17, primary visual cortex
18	Area 18 } secondary visual cortex
19	Area 19
20	Sulcus calcarinus

Fig. 108. The neuronal connections in the retinogeniculocortical projection. The position of tracts and nuclei corresponds to that in Figure 107. The infracalcarine part of area 17 is *shaded*

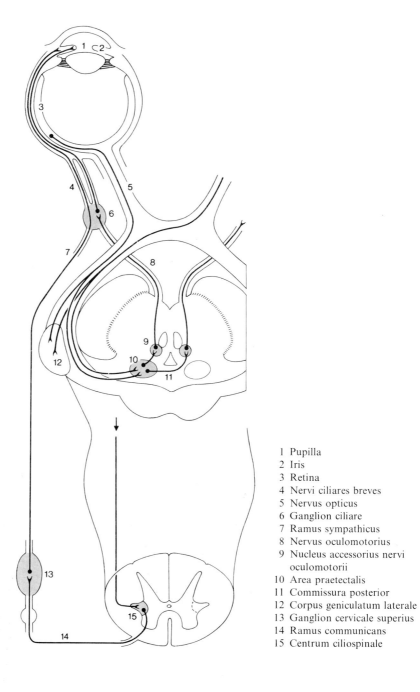

1 Pupilla
2 Iris
3 Retina
4 Nervi ciliares breves
5 Nervus opticus
6 Ganglion ciliare
7 Ramus sympathicus
8 Nervus oculomotorius
9 Nucleus accessorius nervi
   oculomotorii
10 Area praetectalis
11 Commissura posterior
12 Corpus geniculatum laterale
13 Ganglion cervicale superius
14 Ramus communicans
15 Centrum ciliospinale

Fig. 109. The visual system II: the neural reflex arcs of the visual system; the pupillary light reflex

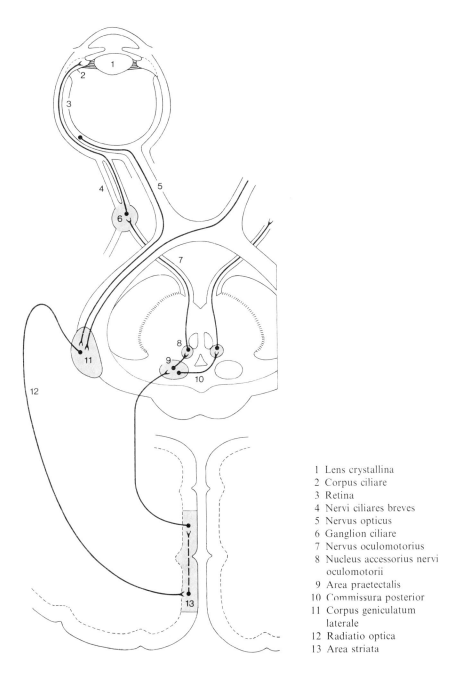

Fig. 110. The visual system II: the neural reflex arcs of the visual system; the accomodation reflex

1 Lens crystallina
2 Corpus ciliare
3 Retina
4 Nervi ciliares breves
5 Nervus opticus
6 Ganglion ciliare
7 Nervus oculomotorius
8 Nucleus accessorius nervi
  oculomotorii
9 Area praetectalis
10 Commissura posterior
11 Corpus geniculatum
   laterale
12 Radiatio optica
13 Area striata

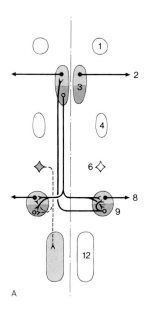

A

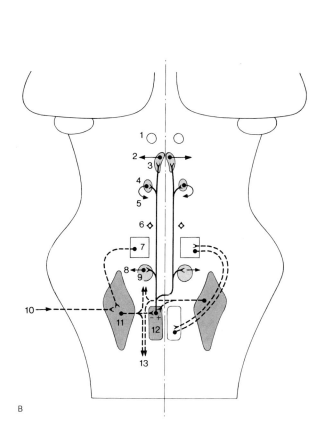

1 Nucleus interstitialis
2 Nervus oculomotorius
3 Nucleus nervi oculomotorii
4 Nucleus nervi trochlearis
5 Nervus trochlearis
6 Formatio reticularis pontis paramedianus
7 Cerebellum
8 Nervus abducens
9 Nucleus nervi abducentis
10 Nervus vestibularis (VIII)
11 Nuclei vestibulares
12 Nucleus praepositus hypoglossi
13 Fasciculus longitudinalis medialis

B

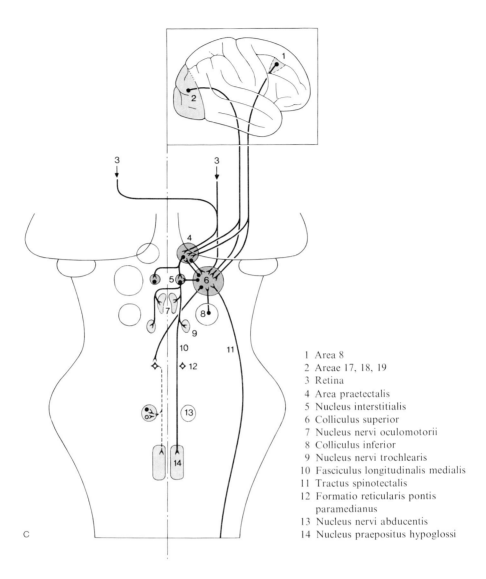

1 Area 8
2 Areae 17, 18, 19
3 Retina
4 Area praetectalis
5 Nucleus interstitialis
6 Colliculus superior
7 Nucleus nervi oculomotorii
8 Colliculus inferior
9 Nucleus nervi trochlearis
10 Fasciculus longitudinalis medialis
11 Tractus spinotectalis
12 Formatio reticularis pontis
   paramedianus
13 Nucleus nervi abducentis
14 Nucleus praepositus hypoglossi

Fig. 111 A–C. The visual system III: the oculomotor pathways. **A** intrinsic connections; **B** ascending pathways; **C** descending pathways

Ascending Reticular System

The Reticular Formation
(Fig. 112)

The area which occupies the central core of the brain stem is known as the reticular formation. Throughout most of its extent this area is occupied by aggregations of loosely arranged cells of different types and sizes, and the fibre systems that pass through its territory are likewise mostly diffusely organised. The term reticular formation refers to the fact that the dendrites of the cells in this area are arranged in bundles that together form a net-like pattern. The traversing fibre systems pass through the interstices of this network. The reticular formation is surrounded by cranial nerve nuclei and relay centres as well as by the long ascending (lemniscal) and descending fibre systems of the brain stem. Caudally the reticular formation is continuous with the substantia intermedia of the spinal cord; rostrally it passes over into the intralaminar nuclei of the thalamus and in certain aggregations of the subthalamic cells among which the zona incerta may be mentioned.

On both cytoarchitectonic and functional grounds the reticular formation can be divided into three longitudinal columns or zones [30]: (1) a median and paramedian zone, which consists of the raphe nuclei, (2) a medial zone which contains many large cells, and (3) a lateral parvicellular zone. Figure 112 shows that a sharp boundary between the medial and lateral zones can only be drawn at the level of the pons and of the rostral medulla oblongata.

The nuclei of the raphe include the nucleus raphes dorsalis, the nucleus centralis superior, the nucleus raphes pontis, the nucleus raphes magnus and the nucleus raphes obscurus (Fig. 112). Studies with the aid of histofluorescence techniques have revealed that many cells in these nuclei show a high content of serotonin. The principal ascending and descending connections originating from the raphe centres are represented in Figure 154.

The medial reticular zone may also be subdivided into a number of centres, which are commonly designated as the nucleus reticularis gigantocellularis, the nucleus reticularis pontis caudalis and the nucleus reticularis pontis oralis. It is important to note that the mesencephalic cuneiform and subcuneiform nuclei as well as a narrow medial strip of the nucleus medullae oblongatae centralis functionally form part of the medial reticular zone.

The cells in the medial reticular zone are provided with long, sparsely branching dendrites that are oriented in the transverse plane. Their axons generally bifurcate into a long ascending and a long descending branch. These branches emit numerous collaterals along their course. The axonal systems of many of the cells in question remain within the confines of the reticular formation and thus serve as links in multisynaptic ascending and descending pathways. However, those of many other elements ascend to the diencephalon or descend to the spinal cord. The afferent systems to the medial reticular zone include (a) a large number of fibres originating from all levels of the spinal cord, (b) fibres or collaterals from relay centres of all sensory cranial nerves, (c) cerebellar afferents, arising mostly from the nucleus fastigii, (d) fibres descending from the hypothalamus and from several limbic forebrain structures, and (e) a strong projection from the premotor area of the cerebral cortex (Figs. 113 and 131). The fibre connections of the medial reticular formation suggest that this area is integrated into both sensory and motor pathways and this has been confirmed by physiological experiments.

The lateral, parvicellular reticular zone lies throughout most of its extent directly medial to the sensory nucleus of the trigeminal nerve. Its most rostral part is formed by the medial and lateral parabrachial nuclei (Fig. 112). In the lower medulla oblongata the bulk of the reticular formation should be considered to form part of the lateral zone [104]. It has been suggested [184] that the axons of the cells in the lateral reticular zone spread medially into the magnocellular medial zone. On this account the lateral zone has been designated as the 'sensory' or 'associative' part of the reticular formation [30]. However, recent investigations [105] have shown that the neurons of the lateral zone are the main source of projections to the bulbar motor nuclei, several of which lie embedded in this zone (Figs. 112 and 132). These neurons probably subserve several bulbar reflexes and are also the recipients of projections descending from higher levels of the brain [105, 141].

The reticular formation contains a few well-defined nuclei that distinguish themselves from the remaining cell groups in this territory by receiving discrete projections from or sending discrete projections to particular centres. Thus the nucleus tegmenti pedunculopontinus, pars compacta (Fig. 112), receives a circumscribed bundle from the globus pallidus, and the nucleus reticularis tegmenti pontis as well as the nucleus funiculi anterioris project massively to the cerebellum [30]. The latter nucleus, which is situated in the lower part of the medulla oblongata, is also known as the nucleus reticularis paramedianus. Another cell mass situated in the lower medulla oblongata which projects massively to the cerebellum is the nucleus funiculi lateralis. Although this cell mass is not of a reticular appearance and is situated beyond the reticular formation it is sometimes referred to as the lateral reticular nucleus.

Stimulation and coagulation experiments have shown that certain areas in the medullary reticular formation play a role in the regulation and control of the circulatory and respiratory systems. These areas exert pressor and depressor effects on heart rate and blood pressure and affect the inspiratory and expiratory phases of respiration. Although the areas involved in these functions are often denoted as 'centres', it should be noted that neither of them is related to a definable anatomical structure. Moreover, they show a considerable overlap.

Ascending Reticular Pathways
(Fig. 113)

After having entered the central nervous system, stimuli gathered by the various kinds of receptors may reach the cerebral cortex either via modality-specific lemniscal systems or via what is called the non-specific afferent or extralemniscal system. Since the reticular formation of the brain stem forms a crucial part of the latter system it is also known as the ascending reticular or, with reference to one of its essential functions, the ascending-reticular activating system. The structural components of this system are (1) the spinoreticular projection, (2) reticular afferents from centres of the various sensory cranial nerves, (3) direct and indirect reticulothalamic fibres, and (4) the 'aspecific' thalamocortical projection. These components are illustrated in Figure 113 and will now be discussed.

1. The spinoreticular projection (Figs. 90 and 96). A large population of cells situated in the intermediate grey of the spinal cord may be characterised as non-specific, because they receive, via interneurons, convergent information from nearly all types of primary afferent fibres [25]. The axons of most of these cells decussate in the anterior white commissure, ascend in the anterolateral funiculus and terminate, either directly, or via one or more synaptic interruptions at spinal levels, in the medial reticular formation. However, a small contingent of these fibres bypasses the reticular core of the brain stem and projects directly to the intralaminar nuclei, which constitute the chief thalamic relay of the ascending reticular system. Although spinal ascending fibres terminate throughout the reticular formation, the majority is distributed to particular levels. One area of maximal termination is situated in the medulla oblongata and coincides with the caudal part of the gigantocellular nucleus and with the rostral part of the central nucleus of the medulla oblongata, a second area of maximal termination is formed by the nucleus reticularis pontis caudalis and a third maximal terminal region is found at the transition from the pons to the mesencephalon [24, 30].

2. Relay centres of all sensory cranial nerves are sources of input to the reticular formation. General somatic afferent stimuli are conveyed by collaterals from the spinal trigeminal nucleus. Visceral afferent impulses are derived from the nucleus of the solitary tract. The vestibular and cochlear nuclei and their pathways have also been reported to project to the reticular formation and the same holds true for the visual and the olfactory system. Optic impulses are mediated by retinotectal and tectoreticular fibre systems. Olfactory impulses probably reach the mesencephalic reticular formation by way of the medial forebrain bundle [175].

3. Reticulothalamic fibres. Fibres preferentially originating from the areas of maximal termination of the spinal afferents ascend through the reticular core of the brain stem and project to the intralaminar thalamic nuclei. This direct reticulothalamic projection is parallelled by indirect ones, consisting of two or more successive neuronal links [184] (Fig. 113).

4. The 'aspecific' thalamocortical projection. The impulses that travelling along the ascending reticular system reach the diencephalic level may be relayed towards the cortex along different paths. It has been recently established [26, 117] that the intralaminar nuclei have a widespread, direct projection to the cerebral cortex. This projection is probably constituted by collaterals of the fibres which connect the intralaminar nuclei with the striatum. Classically cortically projecting thalamic nuclei are way stations in other ascending reticular paths. It is known that several of these 'specific' nuclei, e.g., the ventral lateral and the lateral posterior nuclei, receive afferents from the reticular formation. These reticular afferents reach the nuclei in question either directly or via the intralaminar cell groups (Fig. 113).

Before closing this synopsis of the ascending reticular system three comments should be made. Firstly, it should be emphasised that although many of the spinal cells that project on the reticular formation receive impulses from various sensory modalities and although a further convergence of sensory impulses occurs at the brain stem level, this does not mean that all of the neuronal units participating in the ascending reticular system are entirely 'non-specific'. Thus it is known that pain and other protopathic stimuli may well be conducted upwards by this system with maintenance of their specificity. The second point to be emphasised is that the ascending and descending reticular systems are by no means independent of each other. Rather, the neural network of the reticular formation allows a considerable interaction between ascending and descending impulses [31]. Thirdly, the ascending reticular system projects not exclusively to the cortex but also to a large number of subcortical centres. The massive thalamostriate system, connecting the intralaminar nuclei with the caudate nucleus and the putamen, has already been mentioned. Other subcortical projections discharge fibres into the zona incerta, the preoptic region, the septum and into various hypothalamic areas [26, 69, 184].

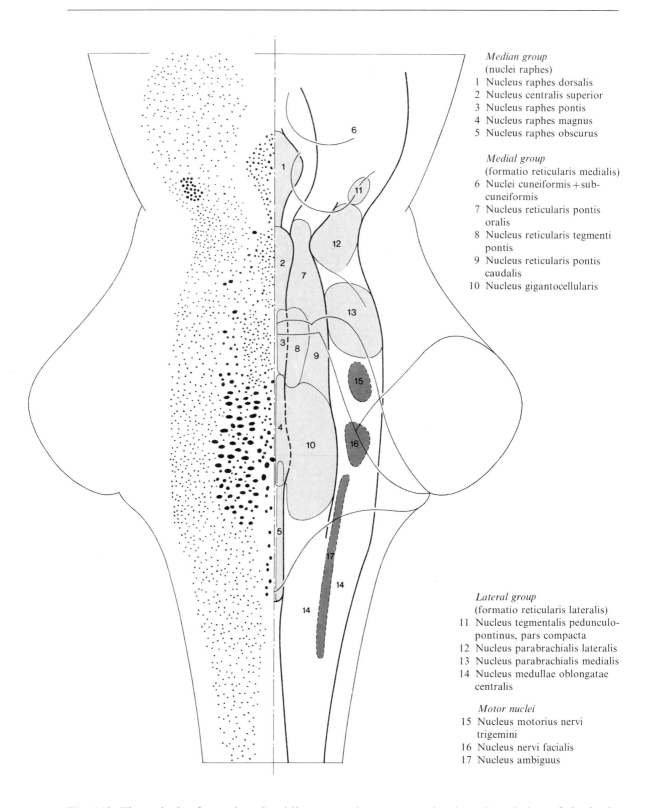

Fig. 112. The reticular formation. Semidiagrammatic representation in a dorsal view of the brain stem. *Left*: cytoarchitecture; *right*: subdivision. The cranial nerve motor nuclei are *darkly shaded*

Median group
(nuclei raphes)
1 Nucleus raphes dorsalis
2 Nucleus centralis superior
3 Nucleus raphes pontis
4 Nucleus raphes magnus
5 Nucleus raphes obscurus

Medial group
(formatio reticularis medialis)
6 Nuclei cuneiformis + subcuneiformis
7 Nucleus reticularis pontis
   oralis
8 Nucleus reticularis tegmenti
   pontis
9 Nucleus reticularis pontis
   caudalis
10 Nucleus gigantocellularis

Lateral group
(formatio reticularis lateralis)
11 Nucleus tegmentalis pedunculopontinus, pars compacta
12 Nucleus parabrachialis lateralis
13 Nucleus parabrachialis medialis
14 Nucleus medullae oblongatae
   centralis

Motor nuclei
15 Nucleus motorius nervi
   trigemini
16 Nucleus nervi facialis
17 Nucleus ambiguus

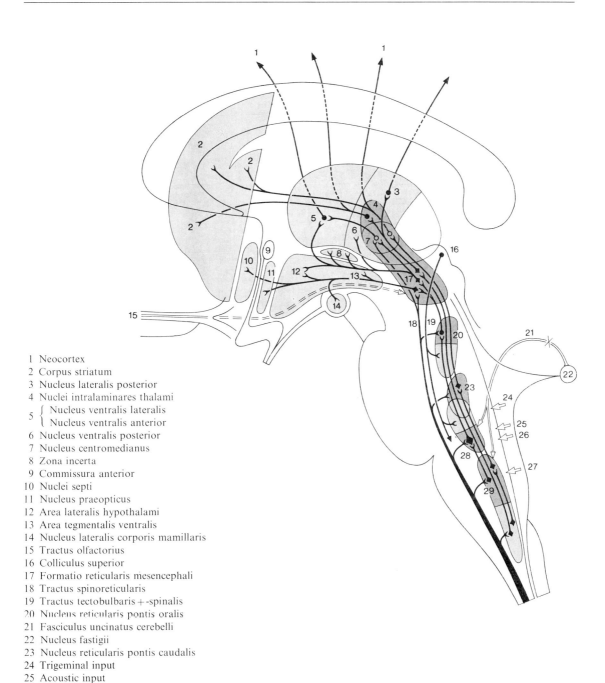

1 Neocortex
2 Corpus striatum
3 Nucleus lateralis posterior
4 Nuclei intralaminares thalami
5 { Nucleus ventralis lateralis
    Nucleus ventralis anterior
6 Nucleus ventralis posterior
7 Nucleus centromedianus
8 Zona incerta
9 Commissura anterior
10 Nuclei septi
11 Nucleus praeopticus
12 Area lateralis hypothalami
13 Area tegmentalis ventralis
14 Nucleus lateralis corporis mamillaris
15 Tractus olfactorius
16 Colliculus superior
17 Formatio reticularis mesencephali
18 Tractus spinoreticularis
19 Tractus tectobulbaris + -spinalis
20 Nucleus reticularis pontis oralis
21 Fasciculus uncinatus cerebelli
22 Nucleus fastigii
23 Nucleus reticularis pontis caudalis
24 Trigeminal input
25 Acoustic input
26 Vestibular input
27 Solitarian input
28 Nucleus gigantocellularis
29 Nucleus medullae oblongatae centralis

Fig. 113. Ascending fibre systems of the reticular formation. For the descending fibres see Figures 131 and 132

Cerebellum
(Figs. 114–120)

Transverse fissures of different depth divide the cerebellum in lobes, lobules and folia. Paramedian sulci, which are deepest in the posterior lobe, separate the vermis from the hemispheres. The surface of the cerebellum is formed by a cortex that presents a uniform, three-layered histological structure throughout its extent. These layers are, passing from superficial to deep, the cell-poor molecular layer, the monolayered Purkinje layer and the granular layer. The profusely branching, flattened dendritic trees of the Purkinje cells extend into the molecular layer, where they are orientated perpendicular to the direction of the transverse fissures. The deepest layer consists of numerous small granule cells. The axons of these cells ascend to the molecular layer where they dichotomise and run parallel to the transverse fissures, through the Purkinje cell dendritic trees with which they make excitatory synapses. In all layers different types of short axon cells are present, which close feed-forward or feed-back inhibitory circuits [67, 197]. The deep cerebellar nuclei to which most of the Purkinje cells project are located in the central white matter close to the ventricular surface.

Afferent, intrinsic and efferent cerebellar connections can be distinguished. Cerebellar afferents enter the cerebellum from the pons in the middle cerebellar peduncle and from the spinal cord and the medulla oblongata in the inferior cerebellar peduncle (Figs. 114 and 115). Cerebellar afferents can be divided into mossy fibres, which terminate on the granule cells of the cerebellar cortex, and climbing fibres, which terminate on the dendrites of the Purkinje cells (Figs. 115 and 118). Both mossy and climbing fibres give off collaterals that terminate in the central nuclei located in the cerebellar white matter. Intrinsic connections consist of the Purkinje cell axons, which connect the cerebellar cortex with the central cerebellar nuclei. Efferent cerebellar connections originate from the central nuclei. Ascending fibres constitute the superior cerebellar peduncle and descending efferents are located in the inferior cerebellar peduncle.

Mossy fibre systems terminate bilaterally in certain cerebellar lobules. Root fibres of the vestibular nerve and secondary vestibulo-cerebellar fibres from the vestibular nuclei terminate in the flocculo-nodular lobe. Fibres from the posterior spinocerebellar tract originate from Clarke's thoracic nucleus and enter the cerebellum through the inferior cerebellar peduncle. The anterior spinocerebellar tract originates from the spinal border cells and passes rostral to the trigeminal root to enter the cerebellum through the superior cerebellar peduncle. Spinocerebellar fibres and fibres from the lateral cuneate nucleus (the arm equivalent of the posterior spinocerebellar tract) terminate both in the anterior lobe and the region immediately behind the primary fissure. On the caudal aspect of the cerebellum they end in the pyramis and the adjoining part of the hemisphere, the gracile lobule (Fig. 116). In both regions fibres from the posterior spinocerebellar tract (leg) terminate ventrally to those from the lateral cuneate nucleus (arm). Reticulocerebellar fibres from the nuclei of the lateral and anterior funiculi in the lower brain stem, terminate in a slightly more extensive region. Pontocerebellar fibres originate bilaterally from the nuclei pontis, which receive a strong, topically organised projection from the cerebral cortex and the nucleus reticularis tegmenti pontis, which in addition receives a recurrent pathway from the central cerebellar nuclei via the descending branch of the superior cerebellar peduncle. Pontocerebellar fibres terminate in all the lobules of the hemisphere. In the vermis they preponderate in declive, folium and tuber and in the uvula [147, 263].

Climbing fibres originate from the contralateral inferior olive and reach the cerebellum via the inferior cerebellar peduncle (Figs. 117 and 118). They show a mediolateral disposition similar to the intrinsic connections between the cerebellar cortex and the central nuclei. The terminal fields of the climbing fibre paths, therefore, are arranged perpendicular to those of the mossy fibre systems. Fibres from the caudal parts of both accessory olives, which receive fibres from the spinal cord, terminate in the entire hemivermis and in the fastigial nucleus. Olivocerebellar fibres from the rostral parts of both accessory olives, which receive spino-olivary fibres and descending fibres from the central grey in the medial tegmental tract, terminate in the pars intermedia of the hemisphere and in the interposed nuclei (nucleus emboliformis and nucleus globosus). Fibres from the principal olive, which receives the central tegmental tract, terminate in the hemisphere and the dentate nucleus [29, 83]. Reciprocal connections exist between the interposed and dentate nuclei and the corresponding parts of the inferior olive [248]. The tegmental tracts can also be considered part of a recurrent

olivocerebellar loop. The superior cerebellar peduncle, which originates from the dentate and interposed nuclei, decussates and terminates in the parvocellular part of the red nucleus, which gives rise to the central tegmental tract, and in the central grey, from which the medial tegmental tract descends towards the inferior olive.

Efferent cerebellar connections include axons of the central nuclei to the vestibular nuclei and direct corticofugal fibres, which terminate in the vestibular nuclei (Figs. 119 and 120).

The latter take their origin from the anterior lobe vermis as Purkinje cell axons that terminate in the lateral vestibular nucleus and from the flocculus and the nodule to the other vestibular nuclei [262]. Central nuclear axons from the fastigial nucleus, some of which cross inside the cerebellum to constitute the uncinate fascicle, terminate bilaterally in the vestibular nuclei and the reticular formation. The ascending branch of the uncinate tract reaches the thalamus, where it terminates in the ventral anterior and ventral lateral nuclei. The dentate and interposed nuclei give rise to the superior cerebellar peduncle which decussates in the mesencephalon. Here fibres of the interposed nuclei terminate in the central grey and on the magnocellular portion of the red nucleus, and fibres of the dentate, in its parvocellular part. Beyond the red nucleus fibres from the superior cerebellar peduncle terminate in the ventral anterior and ventral lateral nuclei [43, 164], which project to the motor and premotor cortex in the frontal lobe. In the thalamus the cerebellar projections partially overlap with those of the globus pallidus. Ultimately each hemivermis is connected bilaterally with the spinal cord through the fastigial nucleus and the vestibulospinal and reticulospinal tracts in the medial longitudinal fascicle. Connections between the hemisphere and the cord from the interposed nuclei include the superior cerebellar peduncle and the rubrospinal tract. The connection starting from the interposed and dentate nuclei comprises the superior cerebellar peduncle, the ventral lateral and ventral anterior nuclei of the thalamus, the motor and supplementary motor cortex and the pyramid. Because the superior cerebellar peduncle and the rubrospinal and pyramidal tracts cross, each hemisphere is ultimately connected with the ipsilateral cord.

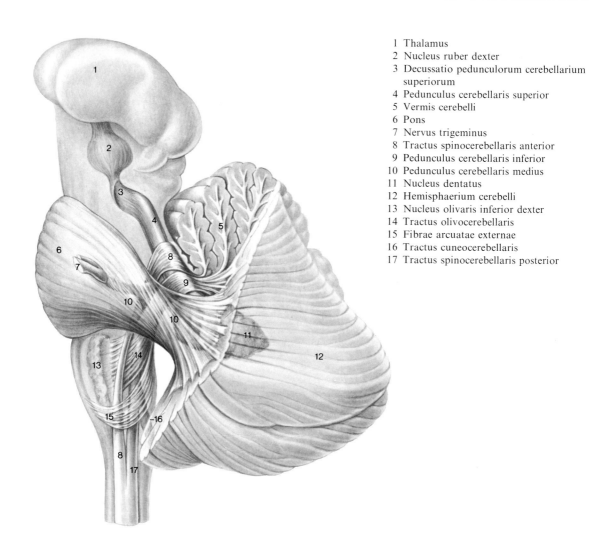

1 Thalamus
2 Nucleus ruber dexter
3 Decussatio pedunculorum cerebellarium
   superiorum
4 Pedunculus cerebellaris superior
5 Vermis cerebelli
6 Pons
7 Nervus trigeminus
8 Tractus spinocerebellaris anterior
9 Pedunculus cerebellaris inferior
10 Pedunculus cerebellaris medius
11 Nucleus dentatus
12 Hemisphaerium cerebelli
13 Nucleus olivaris inferior dexter
14 Tractus olivocerebellaris
15 Fibrae arcuatae externae
16 Tractus cuneocerebellaris
17 Tractus spinocerebellaris posterior

△

Fig. 114. The pedunculi of the cerebellum in a lateral view (3/2 ×)

Fig. 115. The afferent connections of the cerebellum I: distribution of the mossy fibre systems ▷

Fig. 116. The cerebellar cortex, unfolded into one plane, showing the fields of termination of the mossy fibre systems: pontocerebellar fibres (*open contours*), spino- and cuneocerebellar fibres (*dotted*) and vestibulocerebellar fibres (*hatched*)

1 Tractus pyramidalis
2 Nucleus ruber
3 Pedunculus cerebellaris superior,
  ramus descendens
4 Tractus rubrospinalis
5 Formatio reticularis pontis
6 Nuclei pontis
7 Pedunculus cerebellaris medius
8 Pedunculus cerebellaris inferior
9 Nuclei centrales cerebelli
10 Nervus vestibularis (VIII)
11 Nuclei vestibulares
12 Fasciculus uncinatus cerebelli
13 Lobus flocculonodularis
14 Formatio reticularis myelencephali
15 Tractus cuneocerebellaris
16 Nucleus cuneatus lateralis
17 Tractus spinocerebellaris anterior
18 Tractus spinocerebellaris posterior
19 Funiculus posterior
20 Cellulae motoriae cornus anterioris
21 Substantia intermedia
22 Radix dorsalis nervi spinalis
23 Nucleus thoracicus
24 "Bordercell" (of anterior horn)

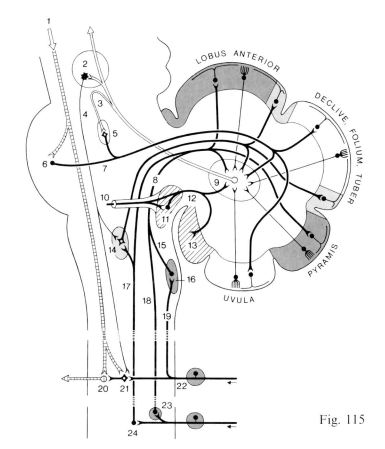

Fig. 115

Li Lingula cerebelli
Ce Lobulus centralis
Cu Culmen
De Declive
Fo Folium vermis
Tu Tuber vermis
Py Pyramis vermis
Uv Uvula vermis
No Nodulus

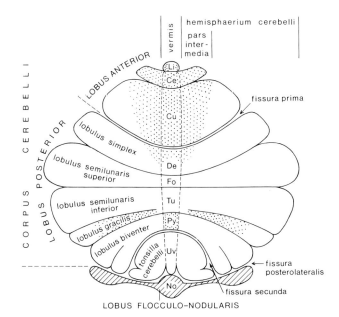

Fig. 116

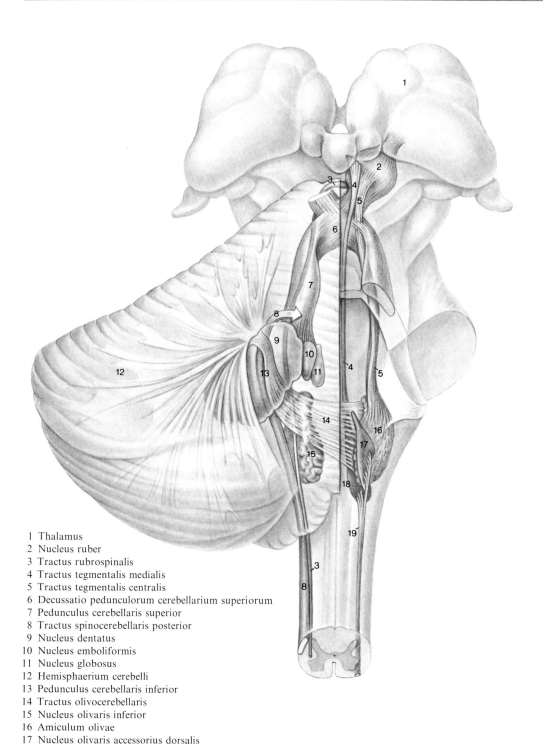

1 Thalamus
2 Nucleus ruber
3 Tractus rubrospinalis
4 Tractus tegmentalis medialis
5 Tractus tegmentalis centralis
6 Decussatio pedunculorum cerebellarium superiorum
7 Pedunculus cerebellaris superior
8 Tractus spinocerebellaris posterior
9 Nucleus dentatus
10 Nucleus emboliformis
11 Nucleus globosus
12 Hemisphaerium cerebelli
13 Pedunculus cerebellaris inferior
14 Tractus olivocerebellaris
15 Nucleus olivaris inferior
16 Amiculum olivae
17 Nucleus olivaris accessorius dorsalis
18 Nucleus olivaris accessorius medialis
19 Tractus spino-olivaris

Fig. 117. The olivocerebellar circuits. Position of tracts and nuclei in a dorsal view (5/3×). The cerebellum was split in the midline and the right half removed

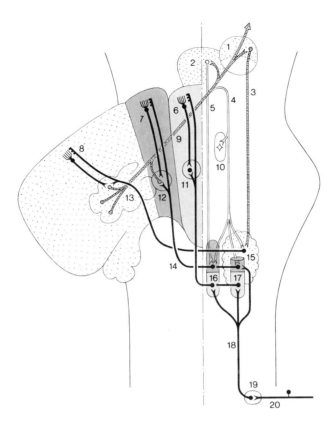

1 Nucleus ruber
2 Griseum centrale mesencephali
3 Tractus tegmentalis centralis
4 Pedunculus cerebellaris superior,
   ramus descendens
5 Tractus tegmentalis medialis
6 Vermis cerebelli
7 Hemisphaerium cerebelli, pars intermedia
8 Hemisphaerium cerebelli
9 Pedunculus cerebellaris superior
10 { Nucleus reticularis tegmenti pontis
   { Nucleus reticularis pontis oralis
11 Nucleus fastigii
12 Nucleus interpositus
13 Nucleus dentatus
14 Tractus olivocerebellaris
15 Nucleus olivaris inferior
16 Nucleus olivaris accessorius medialis
17 Nucleus olivaris accessorius dorsalis
18 Tractus spino-olivaris
19 Nucleus proprius
20 Radix dorsalis nervi spinalis

Fig. 118. The afferent connections of the cerebellum II: the climbing fibres from the inferior olive and the associated circuits

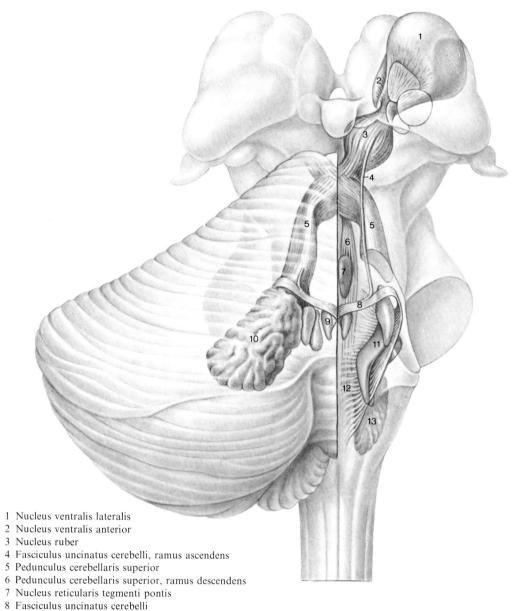

1 Nucleus ventralis lateralis
2 Nucleus ventralis anterior
3 Nucleus ruber
4 Fasciculus uncinatus cerebelli, ramus ascendens
5 Pedunculus cerebellaris superior
6 Pedunculus cerebellaris superior, ramus descendens
7 Nucleus reticularis tegmenti pontis
8 Fasciculus uncinatus cerebelli
9 Nucleus fastigii
10 Nucleus dentatus
11 Nuclei vestibulares
12 Formatio reticularis myelencephali
13 Nucleus olivaris inferior

Fig. 119. The efferent connections of the cerebellum. Position of tracts and nuclei in a dorsal view (5/3 ×). The cerebellum was split in the midline and the right half removed

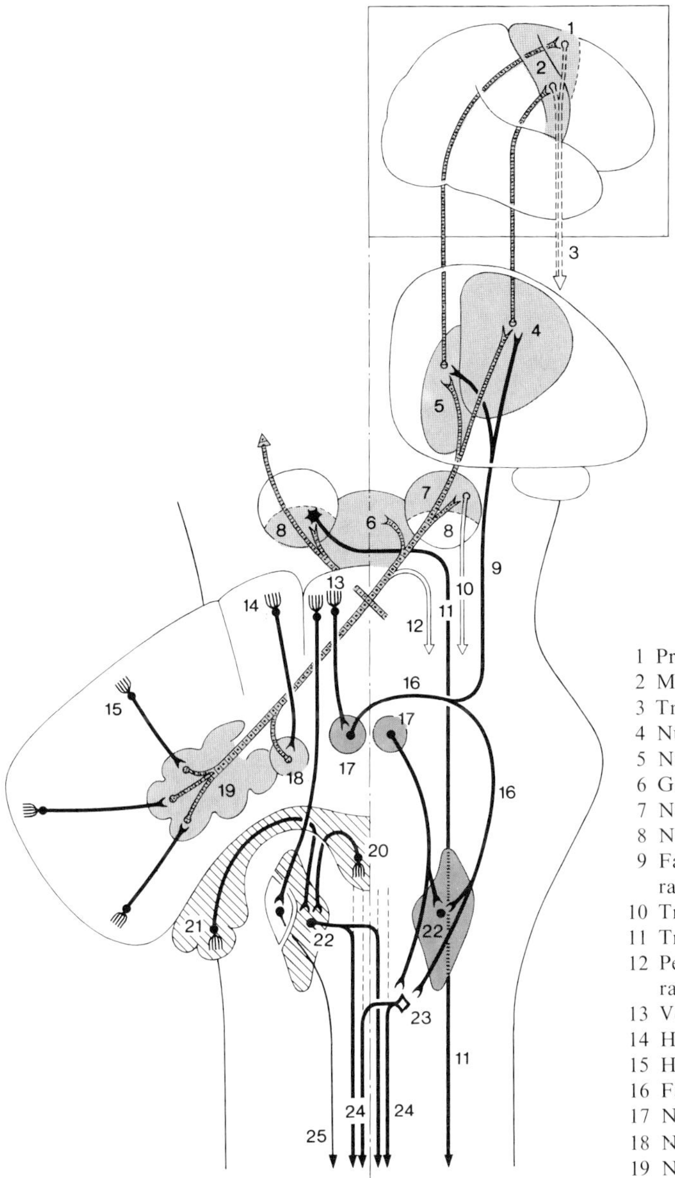

1 Premotor cortex (area 6)
2 Motor cortex (area 4)
3 Tractus pyramidalis
4 Nucleus ventralis lateralis
5 Nucleus ventralis anterior
6 Griseum centrale mesencephali
7 Nucleus ruber, pars parvocellularis
8 Nucleus ruber, pars magnocellularis
9 Fasciculus uncinatus cerebelli,
    ramus ascendens
10 Tractus tegmentalis centralis
11 Tractus rubrospinalis
12 Pedunculus cerebellaris superior,
    ramus descendens
13 Vermis cerebelli
14 Hemisphaerium cerebelli, pars intermedia
15 Hemisphaerium cerebelli
16 Fasciculus uncinatus cerebelli
17 Nucleus fastigii
18 Nucleus interpositus
19 Nucleus dentatus
20 Nodulus   ⎫
              ⎬ Lobus flocculonodularis
21 Flocculus ⎭
22 Nuclei vestibulares
23 Formatio reticularis myelencephali
24 Fasciculus longitudinalis medialis
25 Tractus vestibulospinalis lateralis

Fig. 120. The efferent connections of the cerebellum

Thalamocortical and Corticothalamic Connections
(Figs. 121–123)

The thalamus is a nuclear complex located in the wall of the diencephalon, caudal to the interventricular foramen. During development, part of the medial wall of the hemisphere adheres to the dorsal thalamic surface (lamina affixa). Consequently the thalamus becomes located in the floor of the central part of the lateral ventricle. Laterally the lamina medullaris externa borders the thalamus against the internal capsule. The reticular nucleus of the thalamus is located between the external medullary lamina and the internal capsule. This nucleus becomes perforated by bundles of thalamocortical and corticothalamic fibres that become detached from the internal capsule and enter the thalamus. Ventral to the thalamus, the reticular nucleus continues in the zona incerta of the subthalamus. Fibres from the superior cerebellar peduncle and the globus pallidus pass through the ventral portion of the external medullary lamina between thalamus and zona incerta to end in the anterior thalamus.

Corticothalamic and thalamocortical fibres that become detached from the corona radiata and enter the thalamus at its rostral and caudal poles and along its dorsal surface are termed the thalamic peduncles. Figure 123 shows that they are located medial to the long corticofugal pathways which descend to the brain stem and the spinal cord. The anterior thalamic peduncle breaks away from the anterior limb of the internal capsule and its fibres form a reciprocal connection with the prefrontal and orbitofrontal parts of the cortex and the gyrus cinguli. The superior and posterior thalamic peduncles diverge from the posterior limb of the internal capsule and their fibres form a two-way connection between the thalamus and the central parietal and occipitotemporal areas. The inferior thalamic peduncle reaches the thalamus at its ventromedial side, medial to the posterior limb of the internal capsule. It contains fibres connecting the thalamus and the orbitofrontal, insular and temporal cortex and the basal prosencephalon. Amygdalothalamic fibres enter the inferior thalamic peduncle from the ventral amygdalofugal pathway (cf. Figs. 136, 137 and 143).

The curved internal medullary lamina divides the thalamus into the medial thalamic nucleus and the ventral and lateral groups of thalamic nuclei. The nomenclature used in this atlas (see also Figs. 24 and 25) is based on WALKER [265] and OLSZEWSKI [195]. In its rostral part the internal medullary lamina encloses the anterior nucleus. The lateral nuclear group includes the pulvinar, the massive caudal pole of the thalamus. The rostral portion of the lateral group tapers and includes the lateral posterior and lateral dorsal nuclei. The ventral group of nuclei extends more rostrally. It is divided into the ventral anterior, the ventral lateral and the ventral posterior nuclei. Caudally the ventral posterior nucleus is replaced by the medial geniculate body. Together with the lateral geniculate body it belongs to the metathalamus. Several small nuclei constitute the midline nuclear group.

Apart from myelinated fibres, the internal medullary lamina contains the cells of the intralaminar nuclei. The most prominent of these is the nucleus centromedianus in the caudal thalamus. The nucleus parafascicularis is located medial to it, around the fibre bundles of the habenulo-interpeduncular tract (the fasciculus retroflexus).

The thalamus and the cortex are reciprocally connected. These connections in the human brain were recently analysed by VAN BUREN and BORKE [257] on the basis of the literature and in particular with reference to a large number of clinical cases with cortical lesions. The anterior nucleus, the recipient of the mamillothalamic tract and of fibres from the fornix, is connected with the cortex of the gyrus cinguli. The medial, ventral anterior and ventral lateral nuclei are connected with the frontal lobe. The medial nucleus is linked to the orbitofrontal and prefrontal cortex. In addition it receives fibres from the amygdaloid nuclei and the hypothalamus by way of the inferior thalamic peduncle. The ventral anterior nucleus is connected with more rostral parts of the frontal lobe (area 6) than is the ventral lateral nucleus (area 4). All regions of both nuclei receive fibres from the cerebellum and pallidothalamic and nigrothalamic connections converge on lateral and medial subdivisions of the ventral lateral and ventral anterior nucleus, respectively [162]. Moreover, intrinsic thalamic pathways to the medial and intralaminar nuclei originate from the ventral anterior nucleus [36]. The ventral posterior nucleus is joined to the postcentral gyrus; fibres of a portion of the ventral nucleus intercalated between the ventral lateral and the ventral posterior nucleus (the nucleus ventralis intermedius) terminating in area 3 on the posterior bank of the central sulcus [90], those of the main portion of the ventral posterior nucleus in the areae 1 and 2 on the convexity of the postcentral gyrus. The medial lemniscus and spinothalamic tract terminate in the ventral posterior nucleus. Taste fibres supposedly terminate in the medial, parvocellular portion of the nucleus, which projects to the parietal operculum and the insula [18].

A different organisation of the thalamocortical projection in a series of rostrocaudally directed columns was recently described for the monkey by KIEVIT and KUYPERS [125]. Each column, which is connected with a particular strip of the cerebral cortex and is oriented obliquely to the internal medullary lamina, contains parts of different thalamic nuclei. Medially located columns, which include the medial parts of the ventral anterior and ventral lateral nuclei, the medial nucleus, parts of the intralaminar nuclei and even a portion of the medial pulvinar, project to the orbitofrontal and prefrontal cortex; more laterally located columns, to more posteriorly located transverse strips in the frontal lobe and the central convolutions.

The lateral nuclear group is connected with the parietal, occipital and temporal association cortex, with the exception of the lateral dorsal nucleus, which resembles the anterior nucleus in its projection. Within this extensive projection area the lateral posterior nucleus is connected with the cortex of the inferior parietal lobule. In experimental investigations of the thalamocortical projection to this lobule in the monkey [120], other nuclei were found to be involved as well. In investigations in other mammals the lateral posterior nucleus was found to be involved in a tecto-thalamico-cortical system conveying visual information [87]. Connections with the temporal operculum (gyri temporales transversi, areae 41 and 42) arise from the ventral portion of the medial geniculate body. Connections of the dorsal, magnocellular portion of this nucleus resemble those of the lateral thalamic nuclei. The connections of the lateral geniculate body with the striate cortex (area 17) in the wall of the calcarine sulcus are more amply documented in the illustrations of the visual system (Figs. 107 and 108).

Intralaminar nuclei project both to the cerebral cortex and to the striatum. The projection to the cortex is sparse and diffuse. The intralaminar nuclei show a topographical relationship with quite wide areas of the cerebral cortex [117]. Massive projections originate from the centromedian nucleus to the putamen and from more rostromedial portions of the intralaminar nuclei to the caudate nucleus [161]. Apart from spinal, reticular, cerebellar and pallidal afferents, the intralaminar nuclei receive projections from frontal areae 6 (to central lateral and parafascicular nuclei) and 4 (to the nucleus centromedianus) [161, 162], and intrinsic thalamic afferents, from the ventral anterior nucleus [36].

The reticular nucleus of the thalamus does not project to the cerebral cortex. Its axons terminate in the thalamic nuclei. Cells of the reticular nucleus receive collaterals of the corticothalamic and thalamocortical fibres passing through it [35, 116, 169].

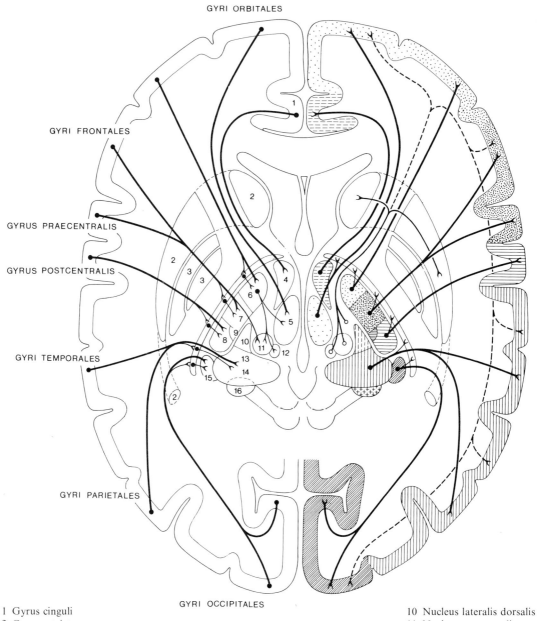

GYRI ORBITALES

GYRI FRONTALES

GYRUS PRAECENTRALIS

GYRUS POSTCENTRALIS

GYRI TEMPORALES

GYRI PARIETALES

GYRI OCCIPITALES

1 Gyrus cinguli
2 Corpus striatum
3 Globus pallidus
4 Nucleus anterior thalami
5 Nucleus medialis thalami
6 Nucleus ventralis anterior
7 Nucleus ventralis lateralis
8 Nucleus ventralis posterior
9 Nucleus ventralis posterior, pars parvocellularis

10 Nucleus lateralis dorsalis
11 Nucleus centromedianus
12 Nucleus parafascicularis
13 Nucleus lateralis posterior
14 Pulvinar thalami
15 Corpus geniculatum laterale
16 Corpus geniculatum mediale

Fig. 121. Connections between the thalamic nuclei and the cerebral cortex I: diagrammatic horizontal section. *Left*: corticothalamic projections; *right*: thalamocortical projections

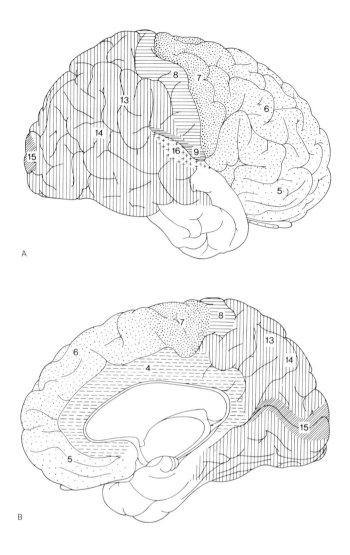

Fig. 122A and B. Connections between the thalamic nuclei and the cerebral cortex II: cortical projection areas of the thalamic nuclei. **A** lateral view; **B** medial view. The shading is the same as that used in Figure 121. For explanation of numbers see also Figure 121

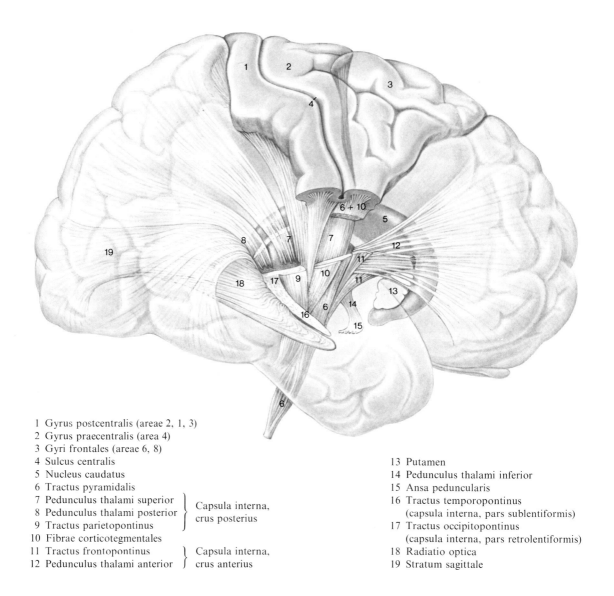

1 Gyrus postcentralis (areae 2, 1, 3)
2 Gyrus praecentralis (area 4)
3 Gyri frontales (areae 6, 8)
4 Sulcus centralis
5 Nucleus caudatus
6 Tractus pyramidalis
7 Pedunculus thalami superior ⎫
8 Pedunculus thalami posterior ⎬ Capsula interna,
9 Tractus parietopontinus   ⎭ crus posterius
10 Fibrae corticotegmentales
11 Tractus frontopontinus   ⎫ Capsula interna,
12 Pedunculus thalami anterior ⎬ crus anterius

13 Putamen
14 Pedunculus thalami inferior
15 Ansa peduncularis
16 Tractus temporopontinus
    (capsula interna, pars sublentiformis)
17 Tractus occipitopontinus
    (capsula interna, pars retrolentiformis)
18 Radiatio optica
19 Stratum sagittale

Fig. 123. Lateral view of the thalamic peduncles and the internal capsule ($1/1 \times$). The proximal part of the corticopontine and corticospinal fibre bundles has been removed to show the thalamic peduncles, which are illustrated as compact bundles for reasons of clarity. The origin of the pyramidal tract in the cerebral cortex has been emphasised (cf. Fig. 124)

Motor Systems

Long Corticofugal Pathways

Projection fibres from deep pyramidal cell layers [19, 119, 156, 234, 269, 270] of the cerebral cortex terminate in an orderly manner in the striatum, thalamus, brain stem and spinal cord. In the depths of the hemisphere together with the thalamocortical fibres they constitute the corona radiata and the internal capsule (Fig. 124). Caudal to the optic tract they come to lie on the ventral surface of the brain stem as the cerebral peduncle. After traversing the cerebral peduncle the corticofugal fibres enter the pons and split up in smaller bundles. The medial and lateral corticopontine divisions of the cerebral peduncle terminate on the pontine nuclei and part of the middle division of the peduncle continues, caudal to the pons, as the pyramidal tract. The majority of the pyramidal tract fibres decussate at the bulbospinal junction to descend in the dorsolateral funiculus of the cord as the lateral pyramidal tract. A varying proportion of the fibres of the pyramidal tract does not decussate, but descends in the wall of the anterior fissure of the cord as the anterior pyramidal tract to midthoracic levels.

Corticostriatal and corticothalamic fibres are also illustrated in Figures 128 and 129. In the brain stem, fibres from the motor cortex (area 4) terminate ipsilaterally in the parvo- and magnocellular red nucleus and the pontine nuclei [143], bilaterally on the lateral reticular formation and certain cranial motor nuclei, and mainly contralaterally on interneurons in the spinal intermediate grey and the motoneurons of the anterior horn. Somatomotor nuclei innervating the extrinsic eye muscles and the visceromotor nuclei do not receive direct fibres from the motor cortex. The motor nuclei of the trigeminal nerve, the dorsal portion of the facial nerve nucleus (muscles of upper facial region) and the nucleus ambiguus are innervated bilaterally. The corticomotoneuronal connections to the ventral part of the facial nucleus (muscles of lower facial region) and the hypoglossal nucleus are crossed [137] (cf. Fig. 132). In the spinal cord bilateral terminations are found on the medial part of the intermediate grey. The main termination includes the lateral portion of the intermediate grey matter and the laterally located motoneurons of the anterior horn [226]. From experiments on animals one may conclude that the termination in the lateral portion of the intermediate grey coincides with the projection of the rubrospinal tract from the contralateral magnocellular red nucleus [142, 148, 149].

Fibres from the supplementary motor area (area 6) and the most rostral part of the sensory cortex (area 3) do not terminate on motoneurons, but contribute to the red nucleus, the basal pontine nuclei, the reticular formation (see Fig. 131) and the intermediate grey [138]. Fibres from the frontal and parieto-occipito-temporal (association) cortex constitute the corresponding corticopontine tracts in the medial and lateral portions of the cerebral peduncle. Apart from terminating in the pontine nuclei, fibres from the frontal (area 8), occipital and temporal lobes terminate in the ipsilateral superior colliculus [143].

The direct corticomotoneuronal fibres represent the crucial pathway for voluntary movement. Moreover, the pyramidal tract serves as the final common path for the contralateral dentate nucleus and the ipsilateral striatal circuit, which converge on the ventral lateral and ventral anterior thalamic nuclei and thus connect with the motor and supplementary motor cortices [165].

The So-called Extrapyramidal System

During the first decades of this century the concept was developed that two independent systems, the pyramidal and the extrapyramidal, converge upon the spinal motor apparatus. Contrary to the direct corticospinal, pyramidal system, the extrapyramidal system was thought to consist of an array of centres, which, together with their emergent fibres, constitute a multisynaptic descending system. Striopallidal, pallidorubral, rubrospinal and reticulospinal pathways were considered to be the principal links in this system. Its highest centre, the striatum, was believed to receive its main input from the thalamus. Experimental hodological studies of the last two decades have conclusively shown that the idea of independently operating pyramidal and extrapyramidal systems has to be abandoned. The striatum and the other structures classically known as extrapyramidal centres are not interconnected in a unidirectional chain-like fashion; rather they constitute, with their emerging fibre systems, a number of interrelated loops or circuits, from which at several points output systems emerge. Interestingly, the pyramidal tract has appeared to be the most prominent of these output systems. Before summarising the salient features of the 'extrapyramidal' circuitry, some of the centres involved, viz. the caudate nucleus, the putamen, the globus pallidus, the subthalamic nucleus and the substantia nigra should be briefly commented upon.

The striatum, i.e. the nucleus caudatus plus the putamen is by far the largest subcortical cell mass of the human brain. The nucleus caudatus is throughout its extent closely related to the telencephalic ventricular cavity. Its large globular head rests on the anterior perforated substance and is anteriorly continuous with the putamen. The latter cell mass is situated medial to the insula and constitutes with the pallidum or globus pallidus the lentiform nucleus, a cone-shaped complex with the apex directed inwards. The putamen constitutes the outer part and the globus pallidus the inner part of the lentiform nucleus. The globus pallidus can be subdivided into a lateral and a medial segment. The anterior limb of the internal capsule separates the caudate nucleus largely from the putamen, whereas the posterior limb of the same structure occupies the space between the lentiform nucleus and the thalamus (Figs. 53, 54 and 127).

Structurally the caudate nucleus and the putamen are identical. They have a homogeneous structure throughout and contain numerous small neurons, among which conspicuous large cells are sparsely scattered (Figs. 57–60). The globus pallidus, which is of diencephalic origin, differs histologically considerably from the telencephalically derived striatal nuclei. This centre is chiefly composed of large, widely spaced, fusiform cells.

The subthalamic nucleus is a conspicuous, large-celled nucleus that is situated in the most caudal part of the diencephalon, dorsomedial to the posterior limb of the internal capsule. Its medial part overlies the rostral portion of the substantia nigra (Figs. 125 and 127).

The substantia nigra is the largest cell mass of the mesencephalon. Lying between the tegmentum and the cerebral peduncle, its most rostral part extends into the diencephalon and closely approaches the globus pallidus. Many of its large polygonal cells synthesize dopamine.

In the ensuing survey of the connections of the striatum and related 'extrapyramidal' centres we will distinguish: (1) a principal striatal circuit, (2) three 'accessory' striatal circuits, (3) input systems and (4) output systems [187] (Figs. 129 and 130).

1. The Principal Striatal Circuit: Cerebral Cortex — Striatum — Globus Pallidus — Thalamus — Cerebral Cortex. Contrary to the views of previous workers it has been established that the whole of the neocortex sends fibres to both the nucleus caudatus and the putamen of the same side and that all parts of these two cell masses receive fibres from the cortex. The arrangement of this corticostriate projection is on a simple topographical basis, although there is some overlap in all dimensions of the termination of fibres from different cortical areas [34, 121].

Efferent fibres from the striatum converge toward the globus pallidus and pass radially through both segments of that structure. During their transit through the globus pallidus these striopallidal fibres emit numerous collaterals that synapse with the pallidal neurons. They then leave the globus pallidus and descend to the substantia nigra (Figs. 125 and 129) [71, 72].

The quantitatively most important efferent system of the striopallidum is the pallidothalamic projection. This projection origi-

nates exclusively from the medial pallidal segment. Its fibres initially constitute two separate bundles, the fasciculus lenticularis and the ansa lenticularis, which merge in Forel's field H, after which they ascend as a single bundle, the fasciculus thalamicus, to the rostral part of the thalamus [185] (Fig. 127). The fibres of this pallidothalamic projection, which is topically organised [126, 136], terminate in the nucleus ventralis anterior and in the nucleus ventralis lateralis of the thalamus. The nucleus ventralis anterior thalami is mainly connected with other thalamic nuclei; however, the nucleus ventralis lateralis has strong connections with areae 4 and 6 of the cerebral cortex.

The existence of the projections just described, which are all topically organised, strongly suggests that information derived from the entire neocortex is processed in the striatum, the globus pallidus and the thalamus, respectively, and then is fed back into the motor and premotor areas of the cerebral cortex.

2a. The First 'Accessory' Striatal Circuit: Striatum — Globus Pallidus — Thalamus — Striatum (Figs. 129 and 130). The striopallidal and pallidal efferent fibres, which form the initial part of this circuit, have already been dealt with. It has been shown that a considerable number of fine fibres leave the fasciculus thalamicus before it reaches the ventral tier thalamic nuclei. These fibres enter the internal medullary lamina and terminate in the centromedian nucleus [185]. As has already been mentioned (cf. Ascending Reticular System), fibres arising from the intralaminar thalamic nuclei traverse the internal capsule and project widely, but in an organised fashion upon both parts of the striatum [161].

2b. The Second 'Accessory' Striatal Circuit: Globus Pallidus — Corpus Subthalamicum — Globus Pallidus. The lateral part of the

172 Functional Systems

globus pallidus projects in a topically organised fashion on the subthalamic nucleus [38, 185] and the latter centre is known to project massively back to all parts of the globus pallidus [177].

2c. The Third 'Accessory' Striatal Circuit: Striatum—Substantia Nigra—Striatum. It has already been mentioned that fibres originating from the caudate nucleus and the putamen traverse the globus pallidus and subsequently descend to the substantia nigra. This strongly developed projection is topically organised [84, 243]. Its fibres, which probably contain GABA, terminate mainly in the external, reticular part of the substantia nigra. The major efferent projection of the substantia nigra is formed by a system of extremely fine axons, which reciprocates the strionigral system described above. Studies with histochemical fluorescence techniques have shown that this system consists of dopaminergic neurons, the cell bodies of which are situated in the pars compacta of the substantia nigra [4].

3. Input Systems. The reticular formation of the brain stem and the cerebellum have a quantitatively very important access to the 'extrapyramidal' circuitry. The reticular formation is one of the principal sources of afferent fibres to the intralaminar nuclei and, as pointed out earlier, the latter project to both the caudate nucleus and the putamen. As regards the cerebellar input, a large number of fibres, originating from the dentate nucleus are distributed profusely to the nucleus ventralis anterior and nucleus ventralis lateralis of the thalamus, i.e., the centres of termination of the most prominent outflow channel of the striopallidum. The areas of termination of the dentatothalamic and pallidothalamic projections have been shown to overlap widely [40, 165]. The cerebellothalamic projection forms part of a circuit, including the following centres: cerebral cortex—pontine nuclei—cerebellar cortex—dentate nucleus—thalamus—motor part of the cerebral cortex. It is noteworthy that this 'cerebrocerebellar loop' shares its thalamocortical part with the principal striatal circuit.

A third important input system to be mentioned here is the mesostriatal serotonergic system. In the striatum large numbers of nerve fibres and terminals occur which contain the putative transmitter serotonin. It has been shown that these fibres and terminals are exclusively derived from one mesencephalic cell mass, the nucleus raphes dorsalis [5, 23, 79] (Fig. 154).

4. Output Systems. Since the main outflow of the striatum and the nuclei related with it converge via the globus pallidus and the thalamus upon the motor cortex, the fibres originating from that cortical area constitute the principal output-channel of all of these nuclei. Prominent among the systems emanating from the motor cortical area is, of course, the motor part of the pyramidal tract, but this area also gives rise to a number of other projections, some of which may well consist of collaterals of the pyramidal axons. Such projections terminate in the ventral lateral and centromedian nuclei [140, 161] of the thalamus, in the subthalamic nucleus [209], the nucleus ruber [143] and to the reticular formation of the brain stem. Several of these pathways feed back into centres included in one of the striatal circuits, thus closing additional 'accessory' loops (Fig. 129).

The remaining output pathways of the extrapyramidal system include pallidohabenular, pallidotegmental, nigrothalamic, nigrotectal and nigroreticular projections. The pallidohabenular fibres originate from the medial pallidal segment and terminate in the lateral habenular nucleus [176]. Via this projection the striatal system has access to the circuitry of the limbic system. The pallidotegmental projection is constituted by fibres that separate from the fasciculus thalamicus and descend towards the mesencephalic tegmentum, where they terminate in the compact part of the pedunculopontine tegmental nucleus [185]. The efferent connections of this nucleus are unknown. The nigrothalamic projection originates from the reticulate part of the substantia nigra. Its fibres are distributed over several thalamic nuclei, among which are the medial and the ventral lateral nuclei [41, 217]. The fibres to the latter cell mass form part of a fourth accessory striatal circuit. As regards the other efferents of the substantia nigra mentioned, it has been recently shown that the reticulate part of this centre sends fibres to the colliculus superior and the reticular formation [82, 106, 218]. The nigrotectal fibres terminate in the deeper layers of the superior colliculus, which are known to give rise to tectoreticular and tectospinal pathways. The tectoreticular fibres project to the mesencephalic and rhombencephalic reticular formation. Since the latter structure is the source of a great number of fibres that descend to the spinal cord there is evidence for the existence of two nigrospinal projections, one via the tectum, the other via the reticular formation. Tectoreticular fibres may well interrelate these two projections (Fig. 129).

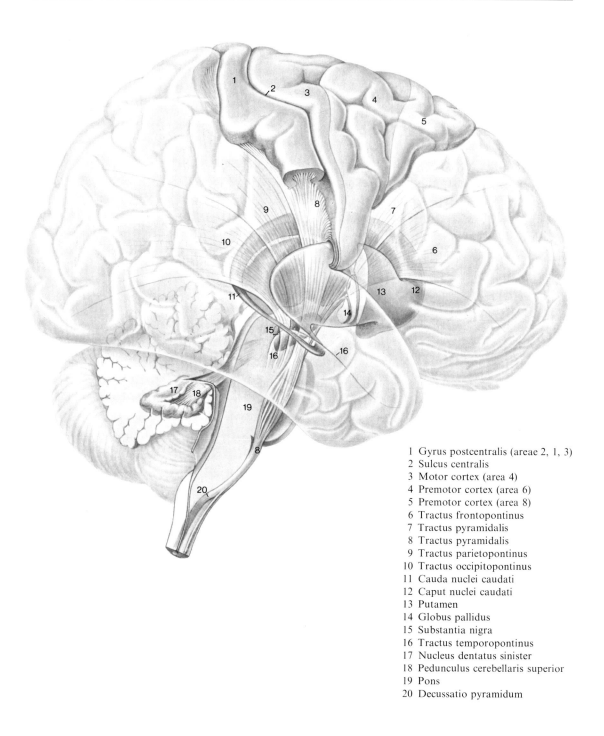

1 Gyrus postcentralis (areae 2, 1, 3)
2 Sulcus centralis
3 Motor cortex (area 4)
4 Premotor cortex (area 6)
5 Premotor cortex (area 8)
6 Tractus frontopontinus
7 Tractus pyramidalis
8 Tractus pyramidalis
9 Tractus parietopontinus
10 Tractus occipitopontinus
11 Cauda nuclei caudati
12 Caput nuclei caudati
13 Putamen
14 Globus pallidus
15 Substantia nigra
16 Tractus temporopontinus
17 Nucleus dentatus sinister
18 Pedunculus cerebellaris superior
19 Pons
20 Decussatio pyramidum

Fig. 124. Pictorial survey of the origin of the pyramidal tract in the cerebral cortex and of the long corticofugal system in a lateral view (1/1 ×). The brain stem and the cerebellum have been cut in the median plane and the right half has been removed, with the exception of the pyramidal tract

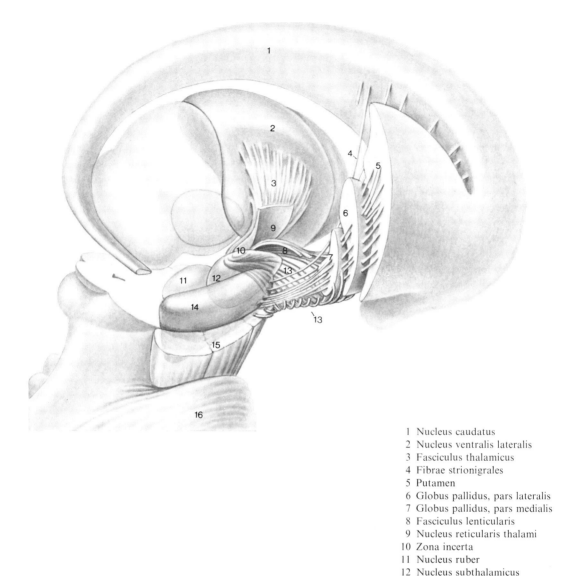

1 Nucleus caudatus
2 Nucleus ventralis lateralis
3 Fasciculus thalamicus
4 Fibrae strionigrales
5 Putamen
6 Globus pallidus, pars lateralis
7 Globus pallidus, pars medialis
8 Fasciculus lenticularis
9 Nucleus reticularis thalami
10 Zona incerta
11 Nucleus ruber
12 Nucleus subthalamicus
13 Ansa lenticularis
14 Substantia nigra
15 Pedunculus cerebri
16 Pons

Fig. 125. The nuclei and fibre bundles of the so-called extrapyramidal system in a lateral view (12/5×). Of the fibres originating from the occipital, removed part of the lentiform nucleus, only the ansa lenticularis is represented

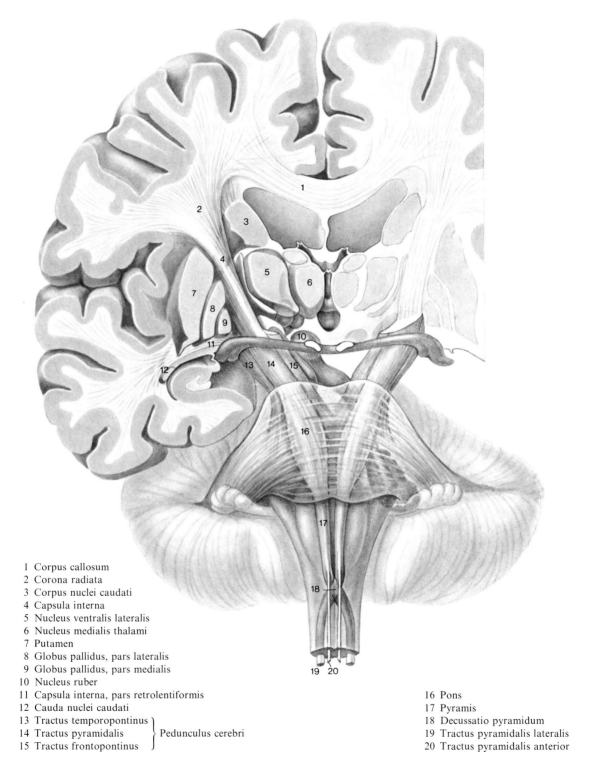

1 Corpus callosum
2 Corona radiata
3 Corpus nuclei caudati
4 Capsula interna
5 Nucleus ventralis lateralis
6 Nucleus medialis thalami
7 Putamen
8 Globus pallidus, pars lateralis
9 Globus pallidus, pars medialis
10 Nucleus ruber
11 Capsula interna, pars retrolentiformis
12 Cauda nuclei caudati
13 Tractus temporopontinus ⎫
14 Tractus pyramidalis   ⎬ Pedunculus cerebri
15 Tractus frontopontinus ⎭

16 Pons
17 Pyramis
18 Decussatio pyramidum
19 Tractus pyramidalis lateralis
20 Tractus pyramidalis anterior

Fig. 126. The long corticofugal fibre system in a frontal view (6/5 ×). The plane of the section shown in this figure coincides with the long axis of the brain stem

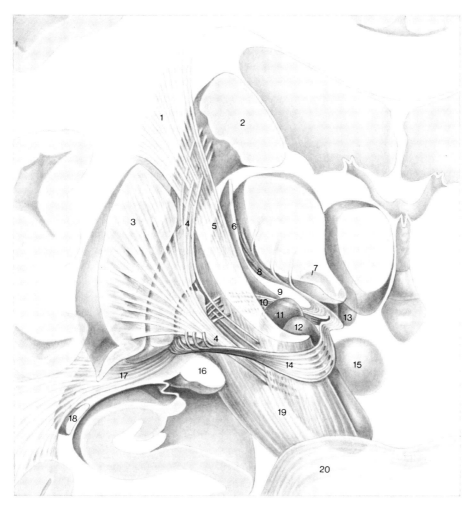

1 Corona radiata	11 Nucleus subthalamicus
2 Corpus nuclei caudati	12 Substantia nigra
3 Putamen	13 Nucleus parafasicularis
4 Fibrae strionigrales	14 Ansa lenticularis
5 Capsula interna, crus posterius	15 Nucleus ruber
6 Nucleus reticularis thalami	16 Tractus opticus
7 Nucleus centromedianus	17 Capsula interna, pars sublentiformis
8 Fasciculus thalamicus	18 Cauda nuclei caudati
9 Zona incerta	19 Pedunculus cerebri
10 Fasciculus lenticularis	20 Pons

Fig. 127. The nuclei and fibres of the so-called extrapyramidal system in a frontal view (12/5×). The fibres originating from the removed frontal part of the lentiform nucleus are not illustrated with the exception of the ansa lenticularis. The plane of the section is the same as in Figure 126

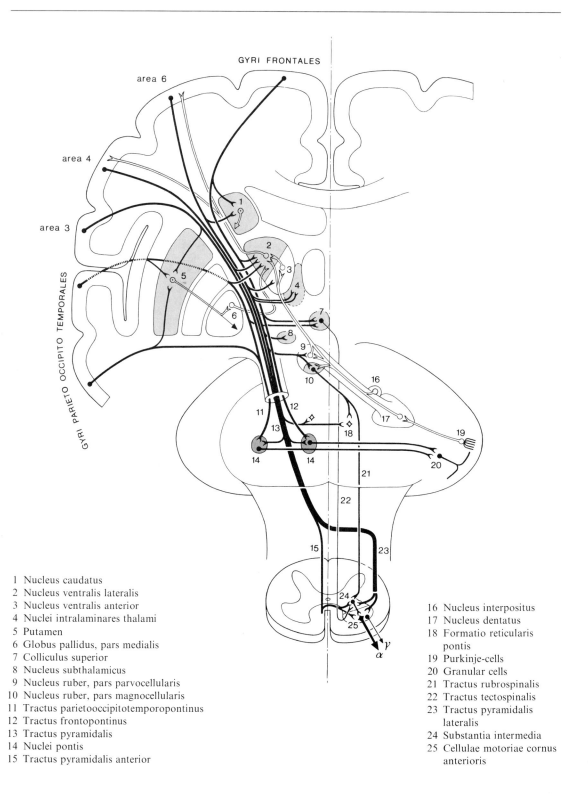

1 Nucleus caudatus
2 Nucleus ventralis lateralis
3 Nucleus ventralis anterior
4 Nuclei intralaminares thalami
5 Putamen
6 Globus pallidus, pars medialis
7 Colliculus superior
8 Nucleus subthalamicus
9 Nucleus ruber, pars parvocellularis
10 Nucleus ruber, pars magnocellularis
11 Tractus parietooccipitotemporopontinus
12 Tractus frontopontinus
13 Tractus pyramidalis
14 Nuclei pontis
15 Tractus pyramidalis anterior

16 Nucleus interpositus
17 Nucleus dentatus
18 Formatio reticularis
    pontis
19 Purkinje-cells
20 Granular cells
21 Tractus rubrospinalis
22 Tractus tectospinalis
23 Tractus pyramidalis
    lateralis
24 Substantia intermedia
25 Cellulae motoriae cornus
    anterioris

Fig. 128. The neuronal connections of the pyramidal system. Feedback pathways are in *open contours*

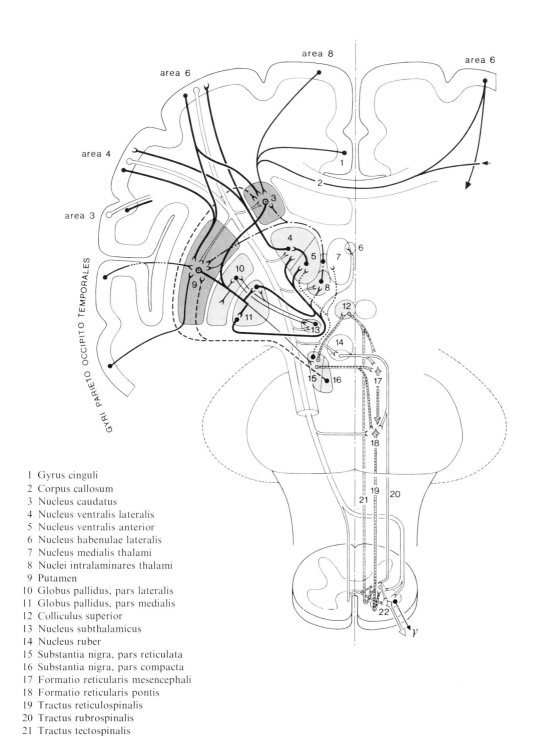

1 Gyrus cinguli
2 Corpus callosum
3 Nucleus caudatus
4 Nucleus ventralis lateralis
5 Nucleus ventralis anterior
6 Nucleus habenulae lateralis
7 Nucleus medialis thalami
8 Nuclei intralaminares thalami
9 Putamen
10 Globus pallidus, pars lateralis
11 Globus pallidus, pars medialis
12 Colliculus superior
13 Nucleus subthalamicus
14 Nucleus ruber
15 Substantia nigra, pars reticulata
16 Substantia nigra, pars compacta
17 Formatio reticularis mesencephali
18 Formatio reticularis pontis
19 Tractus reticulospinalis
20 Tractus rubrospinalis
21 Tractus tectospinalis
22 Cellulae motoriae cornus anterioris

Fig. 129. The main and accessory circuits of the so-called extrapyramidal system. The pyramidal output of the system is added in *open contours*

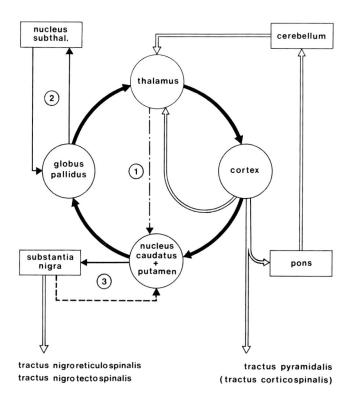

Fig. 130. Summary of the so-called extrapyramidal system. The *bold arrows* represent the main extrapyramidal circuit; the *numbers* indicate the *three accessory circuits described in the text*

Descending Reticular Systems

Descending Pathways and the Medial Reticular Formation (Fig. 131)

For the sake of simplicity we will gather under this heading the reticulospinal tracts and certain descending pathways that impinge upon the cells of origin of these tracts. It should be appreciated that the reticular neurons that project to the spinal cord are influenced by many other afferents (see p. 144) and that the descending parts of the reticular formation cannot be sharply separated from the ascending parts. Within the neural network of the reticular formation there is widespread interaction between ascending and descending impulses [30, 31].

The reticulospinal tracts comprise a pontospinal and a bulbospinal system. The former consists almost exclusively of ipsilateral, the latter, of both crossed and uncrossed fibres. The pontospinal tract originates from the nucleus reticularis pontis caudalis and from the caudal part of the nucleus reticularis pontis oralis. It descends the length of the spinal cord in the anterior funiculus. Its fibres terminate in the anteromedial part of the intermediate substance. The bulbospinal tract, which arises largely from the nucleus gigantocellularis, also extends throughout the length of the spinal cord. Its fibres descend in the anterior part of the lateral funiculus and terminate in the central and dorsolateral parts of the spinal intermediate substance. Both reticulospinal systems act, via interneurons, on alpha as well as gamma motoneurons.

The quantitatively most important input to the reticulospinal neurons is constituted by fibres originating from the cerebral cortex. These fibres, which travel by way of the corticotegmental part of the pyramidal tract, are distributed bilaterally in the reticular formation. The investigations of KUYPERS and his group [42, 139, 141] have shown that the cortical afferents to the medial reticular formation originate mainly from the premotor area. In addition to the medial reticular formation of the lower brain stem, the mesencephalic reticular formation also receives a large number of corticofugal fibres. The mesencephalic reticular formation does not give rise to direct reticulospinal fibres, but it is known that this area contains numerous neurons that project to the pontine and medullary parts of the medial reticular formation [68], thus forming links in an indirect reticulospinal pathway. The mesencephalic reticular formation also receives several fibre systems descending from limbic forebrain structures. These fibre systems include descending constituents of the medial forebrain bundle (Fig. 131), the mamillotegmental tract and the stria medullaris-tractus habenulointerpeduncularis (Fig. 141 B) [178, 179]. Among the many fibre systems converging upon the lower part of the medial reticular formation (cf. p. 144 and Fig. 113), those originating from the cerebellum should be especially mentioned. These fibre systems originate in the nucleus fastigii and pass with the crossed and direct fastigiobulbar bundles to the reticular formation, where they terminate primarily in the nucleus gigantocellularis [15].

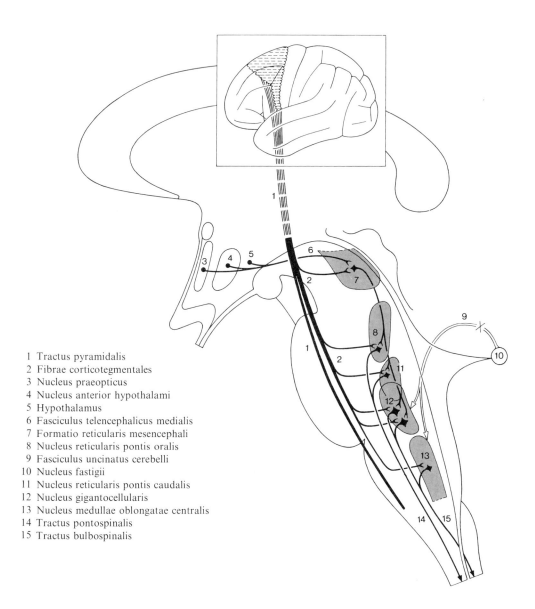

1 Tractus pyramidalis
2 Fibrae corticotegmentales
3 Nucleus praeopticus
4 Nucleus anterior hypothalami
5 Hypothalamus
6 Fasciculus telencephalicus medialis
7 Formatio reticularis mesencephali
8 Nucleus reticularis pontis oralis
9 Fasciculus uncinatus cerebelli
10 Nucleus fastigii
11 Nucleus reticularis pontis caudalis
12 Nucleus gigantocellularis
13 Nucleus medullae oblongatae centralis
14 Tractus pontospinalis
15 Tractus bulbospinalis

Fig. 131. Descending fibre systems of the medial reticular formation. For the ascending fibres see Figure 113

Descending Pathways and the Lateral Reticular Formation (Fig. 132)

The small cells in the lateral part of the reticular formation give rise to relatively short ascending and descending axons which together form a propriobulbar system. The fibres of this system are distributed to the branchiomotor nuclei and to the nucleus of the hypoglossal nerve [104, 105]. These fibres and their parent cells interconnect the afferent components of certain cranial nerves with the efferent system of the lower brain stem, thus constituting links in the various bulbar reflex pathways. However, fibres originating from higher levels of the brain also terminate on the cells of the lateral reticular formation. Prominent among these are cortical fibres, arising from the contralateral motor area (fibrae corticotegmentales), and mesencephalic fibres, arising from the contralateral red nucleus. According to KUYPERS [141] these two fibre contingents constitute, together with the lateral reticular interneurons and the bulbar motoneurons, the supraspinal part of a functional system that is implicated in the control of fine, differentiated movements. A certain proportion of the corticofugal fibres forming part of this system bypasses the reticular interneurons and acts directly on the motoneurons.

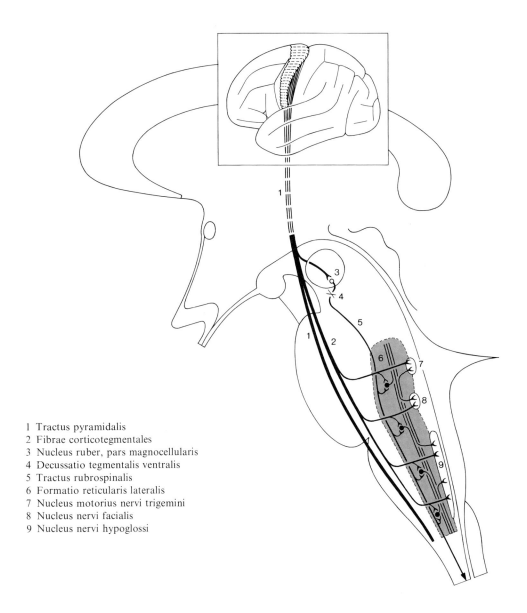

1 Tractus pyramidalis
2 Fibrae corticotegmentales
3 Nucleus ruber, pars magnocellularis
4 Decussatio tegmentalis ventralis
5 Tractus rubrospinalis
6 Formatio reticularis lateralis
7 Nucleus motorius nervi trigemini
8 Nucleus nervi facialis
9 Nucleus nervi hypoglossi

Fig. 132. Descending fibre systems of the lateral reticular formation

Olfactory and Limbic Systems

Certain territories of the diencephalon, the telencephalon and the mesencephalon are structurally and functionally so closely interrelated that they may be considered a single functional complex, which has been designated as the limbic system. At the diencephalic level this system is represented by the hypothalamus; its telencephalic components include the preoptic and septal regions, the hippocampus and some adjacent cortical areas, and the amygdala. The midbrain area of the limbic system is formed by a number of cell masses all of which lie in or close to the median plane. In the present section an attempt will be made to survey the structure and fibre connections of all of these territories. Brief consideration will also be given to the olfactory system, which is intimately related to some components of the limbic system. Indeed, an earlier generation of neuroanatomists considered most of the structures here referred to as limbic, as forming parts of the rhinencephalon. The intricacy of the relationships to be dealt with require, so far as the illustrations are concerned, a three-step procedure: Figure 133 presents the various moieties of the limbic system and their fibre connections in an extremely schematised fashion. This figure will serve as an introductory key diagram. In Figure 134 the major limbic conduction channels are shown semidiagrammatically. This figure is intended as a link between the key diagram and the Figures 137–148, which show the limbic structures and connections in greater detail. Before commencing a concise appraisal of the limbic system two general remarks should be made. First, the literature on the system to be dealt with has grown during the last decennium so overwhelmingly that any attempt at completeness had to be abandoned. Secondly, as in previous sections, with regard to the fibre connections we have relied heavily on the published results of experimental work on laboratory animals. It is by no means unlikely that several or even many of the hodological data presented, in fact do not apply to the human brain, the more so since (1) most experimental studies of limbic pathways have been carried out on rats rather than on primates and (2) it is known that certain limbic structures show considerable interspecific differences [241, 272].

The *hypothalamus* encompasses the most ventral part of the diencephalon, where it forms the floor and a part of the lateral walls of the third ventricle (Fig. 135). Its upper boundary is marked at the ventricular side by a shallow groove, the sulcus hypothalamicus. Caudally the hypothalamus passes gradually over into the periventricular and tegmental grey of the mesencephalon. It is, however, customary to define the posterior margin of the hypothalamus as a vertical plane passing just caudal to the mamillary bodies. The latter are paired small eminences located at the basal side of the brain. The rostral boundary of the hypothalamus coincides with a vertical plane passing from the foramen of Monro to the middle of the optic chiasm. The infundibular stalk, which is situated directly posterior to the optic chiasm, connects the funnel-shaped rostroventral part of the hypothalamus with the pituitary gland.

Within the hypothalamus three mediolaterally arranged zones can be recognised [52]: a periventricular, a medial and a lateral zone. The periventricular zone consists of a few layers of small cells arranged parallel to the ventricular surface. These layers alternate with thin sheets of fine, mostly unmyelinated fibres. The nucleus infundibularis, a cell mass situated in the most basal part of the hypothalamus, may be considered as a derivative of the periventricular zone. The medial zone, which is relatively cell rich, contains a number of more or less individualised cell masses. The latter are usually placed in three groups, an anterior, an intermediate and a posterior group. The anterior group is formed by the rather ill-defined anterior nucleus and by the distinct, magnocellular supraoptic and paraventricular nuclei. The intermediate group consists of the dorsomedial and ventromedial nuclei, cell masses which are poorly delimited from each other. The posterior group includes the medial, intermediate and lateral mamillary nuclei and the diffuse posterior nucleus. The latter nucleus, which contains numerous scattered large cells, is caudally continuous with the periventricular and tegmental grey of the midbrain. The lateral hypothalamic zone is partly separated from the medial zone by the postcommissural fornix, a large bundle connecting the hippocampal formation with the mamillary body (Figs. 134 and 135). The medial surface of the internal capsule and of the subthalamic region form the lateral boundary of the lateral hypothalamic zone. Caudally this zone passes imperceptibly over into the mesencephalic ventral tegmental area; rostrally it is continuous with the lateral preoptic area. Although the lateral hypothalamic zone contains a few local condensations of cells, most of its territory is occupied by a diffuse neuronal matrix known as the lateral hypothalamic area.

The *preoptic region* flanks the rostral-most part of the third ventricle, constituting a rather narrow vertical strip of tissue that extends from the anterior commissure to the rostral part of the optic chiasma. Although this region is of telencephalic origin, it is closely related structurally to the hypothalamus. The three rather poorly differentiated cell masses present in it, i.e., the preoptic periventricular nucleus, the medial preoptic nucleus and the lateral preoptic nucleus, may be considered rostral extensions of the three hypothalamic cell zones.

The *septal region* (also: septum verum or precommissural septum) forms part of the medial wall of the cerebral hemispheres. It is situated directly rostral to the lamina terminalis within the paraterminal gyrus. Dorsally it is bordered by the corpus callosum, rostrally, by the precommissural portion of the hippocampus and caudally, by the anterior commissure and the preoptic region. Ventrolaterally it borders on the nucleus accumbens septi, a large cell mass that in location and function occupies a position intermediate between the limbic and striatal or 'extrapyramidal' systems. Contrary to the prevailing opinion, the septal region is well developed in the human brain [6]. It contains a number of rather poorly individualised cell groups, among which the medial and lateral septal nuclei may be mentioned. The ventromedial part of the septum is occupied by an aggregation of large cells which forms the medial or septal limb of what is known as the nucleus of the diagonal band of Broca. The lateral or tubercular limb of this nucleus extends caudolaterally along the ventral surface of the hemisphere and marks the caudal boundary of the olfactory tubercle. As its name implies this nucleus is embedded in a fibre bundle, the diagonal band of Broca.

The so-called *limbic midbrain area* [179] encompasses two groups of nuclei both of which occupy a paramedian position (Fig. 137). The first group consists of the ventral tegmental area of Tsai, a poorly defined cell mass that is rostrally continuous with the lateral hypothalamic area and of the interpeduncular nucleus. The second group is composed of the ventral part of the central grey substance, the dorsal raphe nucleus, the superior central nucleus (of Bechterew) and the dorsal tegmental nucleus (of Gudden).

Experimental hodological studies have shown that all of the structural entities dealt with are interconnected by shorter and longer ascending and descending fibres. Taken together these fibres constitute one large functional system, which NAUTA [182, 183] has designated as the "limbic system — midbrain circuit". Schematising somewhat it may be stated that the septal, preoptic and anterior hypothalamic areas form the rostral pole of this circuit, whereas the paramedian midbrain area represents its caudal pole. The hypothalamus may be characterised as a nodal way station interposed between these rostral and caudal poles. Two large telencephalic parts of the limbic system, namely the amygdala and the hippocampal formation, as well as the olfactory system are reciprocally connected with the rostral pole of the circuit (Figs. 133 and 134). These structures and their fibre connections will be dealt with below. The caudal pole of the circuit may be considered as a paramedian subdivision of the brain stem reticular formation [69, 183]. The centres forming this pole are to a large extent integrated into both ascending and descending pathways. The ascending pathways connect the lower parts of the reticular formation and the visceral sensory centres situated in the caudal part of the medulla oblongata with the hypothalamus. The descending pathways convey impulses from the hypothalamus to the visceral and somatic motor centres in the brain stem and spinal cord. Focussing now on the hypothalamus, it should be emphasised that this centre, apart from its bidirectional linkages with the various parts of the limbic forebrain-midbrain continuum, entertains several other important functional connections. Among these the following four may be mentioned:

1) The lateral preoptico-hypothalamic zone is reciprocally connected with the medial and certain midline nuclei of the dorsal thalamus [183].

2) The same zone receives a direct input from the orbitofrontal part of the neocortex [181] (Fig. 141A).

3) The mamillary body, which is situated in the caudobasal part of the hypothalamus, receives a large projection from the hippocampal formation and sends most of its efferents to the anterior nucleus of the thalamus. These two connections form part of a closed hippocampo-mamillo-thalamo-cingulo-hippocampal system known as the circuit of Papez (Figs. 134 and 147) [205].

4) The effector mechanism of the hypothalamus includes, apart from fibre systems descending to the brain stem and spinal cord, two hypothalamo-hypophyseal pathways. By way of one of these, the partly neural and partly humoral tubero-infundibulo-hypophyseal system, the hypothalamus controls the production of the various hormones of the anterior pituitary (Fig. 135).

Most fibres that interconnect the rostral and caudal poles of the limbic forebrain-midbrain continuum traverse the hypothalamus. The descending limb of this transhypothalamic projection is, however, supplemented by a notable dorsal conducting route that bypasses the hypothalamus. This route, which is synaptically interrupted in the epithalamic habenular nuclei, is formed by the habenulopetal stria medullaris and the habenulofugal habenulointerpeduncular tract (Fig. 141 B).

After this introductory survey of the circuitry of the central part of the limbic system (Fig. 133), brief consideration will be given to some of the major conduction channels involved in this circuitry.

The *medial forebrain bundle* (Figs. 134, 137, 140 and 141A) may be considered the central longitudinal pathway of the limbic forebrain-midbrain continuum. It is an assemblage of loosely arranged, mostly thin fibres which extends from the septal area to the tegmentum of the midbrain. It traverses the lateral hypothalamic area, the scattered neurons of which are sometimes collectively designated as the bed nucleus of the medial forebrain bundle. The bundle is bidirectional and contains, apart from direct septo-mesencephalic and mesencephalo-septal fibres, a variety of shorter ascending and descending links. Some of its components are diagrammatically represented in Figures 140 and 141 A, and may be documented as follows.

Ascending components:

a) Axons originating from rostral pontine neurons, which terminate throughout the ventromedial nucleus of the hypothalamus. Most of these neurons are located in the dorsal nucleus of the lateral lemniscus [159].

b) Fibres originating from the dorsal tegmental nucleus which via the mamillary peduncle pass to the hypothalamus and then enter the medial forebrain bundle to spread to the lateral preopticohypothalamic area and to the medial septal nucleus [173, 184].

c) Fibres that pass from the ventral tegmental area and from the lateral preopticohypothalamic zone to the septal nuclei [252]. The fibres originating from the hypothalamus reciprocate the massive septohypothalamic component of the medial forebrain bundle [183].

d) Fibres arising from the ventromedial nucleus of the hypothalamus which pass via the medial forebrain bundle to the preoptic region and to the ventral part of the lateral septum [223].

e) Fibres arising from the anterior hypothalamic area which pass through the preoptic region and distribute in the lateral part of the septum [48].

f) Fibres that ascend from the lateral preoptic area to the septum [238].

g) Dopaminergic, noradrenergic as well as serotonergic fibres that connect a number of brain stem nuclei with a variety of prosencephalic structures (see Figs. 151–154).

Descending components:

a) Fibres that pass from the posterior orbitofrontal cortex to the lateral preopticohypothalamic zone [181].

b) Fibres originating from the nucleus of the diagonal band of Broca which terminate in the lateral hypothalamic and ventral tegmental areas [47], as well as in the mamillary body [167].

c) Fibres connecting the dorsal part of the septum with the lateral preopticohypothalamic zone [167].

d) Septal efferents that extend to the ventral tegmental area and to the nucleus centralis superior [179].

e) A massive projection from the septum to the preoptic region [238].

f) Fibres passing from the transition region between the lateral preoptic and lateral hypothalamic areas to the locus coeruleus [238].

g) Fibres originating from the medial preoptic nucleus which pass to most hypothalamic nuclei, to several centres belonging to the limbic midbrain area, including the central grey substance, the ventral tegmental area and the raphe nuclei, and to the mesencephalic reticular formation [47].

h) Fibres that connect the medial preoptic nucleus with the infundibular nucleus [47, 129, 238].

i) Efferents from the anterior hypothalamic area which terminate in the dorsomedial, ventromedial and infundibular nuclei of the hypothalamus, in the ventral tegmental area, the dorsal raphe nucleus, the central grey substance and in the mesencephalic reticular formation. The cells of the paraventricular nucleus project to many of the same areas as do those of the anterior hypothalamic area [48].

k) Fibres originating from the ventromedial nucleus of the hypothalamus which spread to the mesencephalic central grey, the ventral tegmental area and the locus coeruleus [223].

The *dorsal longitudinal fasciculus of Schütz* is, much like the medial forebrain bundle, a composite system consisting of thin ascending and descending fibres. This fascicle extends from the posterior part of the hypothalamus to the caudal medulla oblongata and occupies over its entire length a periventricular position. Most of the ascending and descending projections contained within the dorsal longitudinal fascicle are synaptically interrupted in either the central grey substance of the midbrain or in the dorsal tegmental nucleus of Gudden. It has, however, been recently established that fibres passing directly from the hypothalamus to the autonomic centres of the lower medulla oblongata and vice versa are also present. The components of the dorsal longitudinal fascicle, which are indicated in Figures 140 and 141 B, may be documented as follows:

a) Fibres that originate from the region of the nucleus of the solitary tract and terminate in the dorsal tegmental nucleus [174].

b) Fibres ascending from the dorsal tegmental nucleus and from the rostral part of the mesencephalic central grey. In the hypothalamus these fibres become part of the fine-fibred periventricular system. They terminate chiefly in the posterior part of the hypothalamus [183].

c) Fibres that arise from the caudal part of the nucleus of the solitary tract and ascend to the dorsomedial and paraventricular nuclei of the hypothalamus, to the bed nucleus of the stria terminalis and to the periventricular nucleus of the thalamus [215].

d) Fibres connecting the paraventricular and posterior hypothalamic nuclei with various autonomic centres of the brain stem and the spinal cord. Terminations have been observed in the accessory oculomotor nucleus of Edinger-West-

phal, the dorsal motor vagus nucleus, the nucleus of the solitary tract, and in the intermediolateral nucleus of the spinal cord [54, 86, 222].

e) Descending fibres originating from the medial and periventricular zones of the hypothalamus which are distributed to the mesencephalic central grey and probably to the dorsal tegmental nucleus [37].

f) The dorsal tegmental nucleus is reported [51] to discharge through the dorsal longitudinal fascicle to the branchiomotor nuclei of V, VII, IX and X, to the visceral motor nuclei of VII (superior salivatory), IX (inferior salivatory) and X, as well as to the hypoglossal nucleus.

The *mamillotegmental tract.* The efferents of the mamillary nuclei constitute a large, compact bundle known as the fasciculus mamillaris princeps. This bundle passes dorsally for a short distance and then splits up into two components, the larger mamillothalamic and the smaller mamillotegmental tract (Figs. 134, 135 and 137). The mamillothalamic tract, which passes to the anterior thalamic nucleus, forms part of the so-called Papez circuit (see above and Fig. 147). The mamillotegmental tract curves caudally into the tegmentum of the midbrain and terminates in the dorsal tegmental nucleus and in the nucleus reticularis tegmenti pontis of Bechterew [53] (Fig. 141 B).

The *mamillary peduncle* receives fibres from the dorsal tegmental nucleus. It passes ventrally and then ascends along the ventral surface of the midbrain to the mamillary body where most of its fibres terminate. Some of its fibres join the medial forebrain bundle and spread to the lateral preoptico-hypothalamic zone and to the medial septal nucleus [173, 184].

It has already been mentioned that the *stria medullaris thalami* and the *habenulointerpeduncular tract* constitute together a dorsal conducting route that is synaptically interrupted in the habenular nuclei. The fibres constituting the stria medullaris assemble in the area behind the anterior commissure and pass along the dorsomedial border of the thalamus to the habenular nuclei (Fig. 137). The habenulointerpeduncular tract descends from the habenular nuclei to the basal region of the midbrain, where part of its fibres terminate in the interpeduncular nucleus (Fig. 137). It has been recently established [94] that the two epithalamic cell masses, i.e., the medial and lateral habenular nuclei, represent mutually isolated processing stations in the dorsal conducting route under consideration (Fig. 141 B). The medial habenular nucleus receives by way of the stria medullaris fibres originating from the medial part of the septum and from the nucleus of the diagonal band of Broca [66, 167]. The efferents of the medial habenular nucleus terminate exclusively in the interpeduncular nucleus [95]. The efferent fibres of the interpeduncular nucleus which pass to the dorsal tegmental nucleus form a further link in the 'medial habenular path'. The 'lateral habenular path' comprises (1) fibres that connect the lateral preopticohypothalamic zone with the lateral habenular nucleus [252]; (2) a massive projection from the medial pallidal segment to the lateral habenular nucleus; these fibres follow diverse routes; however, the rostral-most ones reach the epithalamic region by way of the stria medullaris [94, 176]; and fibres originating from the lateral habenular nucleus which descend in the habenulointerpeduncular tract, bypass the interpeduncular nucleus and terminate in various mesencephalic centres, including the compact part of the substantia nigra, the central grey substance, the dorsal raphe and superior central nuclei and the mesencephalic reticular formation [1, 95]. It may be concluded that via this 'lateral habenular path' the extrapyramidal system has access to the circuitry of the limbic and reticular systems. Moreover, the pallido-ha-

benulo-nigral loop forms part of a further 'accessory extrapyramidal circuit' (see p. 168).

Hypothalamo-hypophyseal pathways (Figs. 135 and 140). The magnocellular nuclei of the anterior hypothalamus, i.e., the supraoptic and paraventricular nuclei, give rise to axons that descend through the infundibular stalk to the posterior lobe of the pituitary. These axons, which form together the supraoptico-paraventriculo-hypophyseal tract, transport colloid droplets containing the hormones oxytocin and vasopressin to the posterior pituitary lobe or neurohypophysis, where they are released into the blood. The cells of the nucleus infundibularis are involved in the control of the secretion of the anterior pituitary hormones. They exert this control by means of regulating hormones that stimulate or inhibit the liberation of the hormones produced in the pituitary. Each of the latter has a corresponding regulating hormone. The regulating hormones pass from the infundibular nucleus along the axons of its constituent cells to the median eminence, where they are released from the axon terminals into the capillaries of the hypophyseal portal system. The latter system forms a vascular link between the infundibulum and the adenohypophysis. It is noteworthy that the median eminence, a conspicuous neurohaemal organ situated in the anterior wall of the infundibular stalk, receives apart from the neurosecretory axons just mentioned several other afferent fibre systems that are thought to be concerned in the release of the regulating hormones. Prominent among these are (1) a dopaminergic pathway from the infundibular nucleus (Fig. 151), (2) a noradrenergic pathway from the brain stem (Fig. 153), and (3) a projection from the ventromedial hypothalamic nucleus [134] (Fig. 140)

It has already been mentioned that two

large telencephalic components of the limbic system, namely the amygdala and the formatio hippocampi are reciprocally connected with the rostral part of the central limbic continuum (Fig. 133). These two structures will now be discussed.

The *amygdala* or *corpus amygdaloideum* is a large nuclear complex situated in the dorsomedial portion of the temporal lobe, where it forms part of the rostromedial and rostrodorsal walls of the inferior horn of the lateral ventricle (Figs. 138 and 139). Ontogenetically, the amygdala is a derivative of the caudal part of the ganglionic eminence, an intraventricular protrusion the rostral part of which gives rise to the corpus striatum. Although the anlage of the amygdala during development is displaced rostroventrally, it remains permanently in direct contact with the striatum. The corpus amygdaloideum is divisible into a series of nuclei which may be separated into two major divisions, a corticomedial nuclear group and a basolateral nuclear group [50, 51] (Figs. 58–61). The corticomedial group includes, apart from a number of smaller cell masses, the cortical amygdaloid nucleus and the medial amygdaloid nucleus. Together the nuclei of this group constitute the dorsomedial part of the complex (Fig. 139). The most prominent subdivisions of the basolateral nuclear group are the lateral amygdaloid nucleus, the basal amygdaloid nucleus and the accessory basal amygdaloid nucleus. A rather small central nucleus is sometimes included as part of the corticomedial nuclear group, but will be regarded here as a separate entity. This nucleus is in proximity with the morphologically most caudal parts of the caudate nucleus and the putamen and like these cell masses it harbours a high content of dopamine [254].

Three large fibre bundles, the lateral olfactory stria, the stria terminalis and the ven-

tral amygdalofugal pathway, connect the amygdala with other parts of the brain (Figs. 134 and 139). The lateral olfactory stria carries secondary olfactory fibres to the cortical and medial amygdaloid nuclei. Its course will be considered below. The stria terminalis emerges from the caudomedial aspect of the amygdala, from where it runs a remarkably long curved course along the medial border of the caudate nucleus to the anterior commissure (Figs. 136 and 139). Immediately dorsocaudal to that commissure it splits up into three components: (1) a precommissural or supracommissural component whose fibres descend in front of the anterior commissure, (2) a commissural component that enters the anterior commissure and (3) a postcommissural component that descends caudal to the anterior commissure (Figs. 137 and 143). The stria terminalis is composed of both amygdalofugal and amygdalopetal fibres. The ventral amygdalofugal pathway is a large assemblage of rather loosely arranged fibres which extends from the amygdaloid complex to the rostral part of the diencephalon. It arises from the dorsomedial part of the amygdala from where it passes medially and somewhat rostrally through the sublenticular regions of substantia innominata and substantia perforata anterior. Some of its fibres pass rostrally to the mediofrontal cortex, others spread in the lateral preopticohypothalamic zone and still others enter the inferior thalamic peduncle to terminate in the medial thalamic nucleus [183] (Fig. 139). Contrary to what its name suggests, the ventral amygdalofugal pathway conducts in both directions.

The afferents of the amygdaloid complex can be grouped into the following four categories: (1) fibres originating from the olfactory bulb and from the olfactory part of the cerebral cortex; (2) fibres arising from the preoptic region and from the hypothalamus; (3) direct afferents from the brain stem and (4) projections from various (non-olfactory) areas of the cerebral cortex. These fibre categories, which have been represented diagrammatically in Figure 142, may be documented as follows:

1a. Secondary olfactory fibres originating from the olfactory bulb pass by way of the lateral olfactory tract to the amygdala where they terminate in the cortical nucleus [219, 253]

1b. The basolateral complex receives, according to POWELL et al. [210] and VALVERDE [256], an indirect olfactory input via a relay in the prepiriform cortex. The existence of a prepiriform-amygdaloid projection has, however, been denied by SCOTT and LEONARD [227].

2a. Fibres originating from the lateral preopticohypothalamic zone pass through the stria terminalis and spread to most amygdaloid nuclei [238].

2b. Other fibres with roughly the same sites of origin and termination as those indicated under 2a travel by way of the ventral amygdalofugal pathway [238].

2c. A system comparable to that mentioned under 2a but originating in addition from the bed nucleus of the stria terminalis was previously described by NAUTA [180] and by COWAN et al. [49].

2d. Neurons located in the ventromedial hypothalamic nucleus project to the amygdala, "probably via a route other than the stria terminalis" [213].

3. Pontine gustatory units located in the parabrachial nuclei project via the ventral amygdalofugal pathway to the central nucleus of the amygdala [190].

4a. A cingulo-amygdaloid connection, originating from area 24, has been reported by PANDYA et al. [203]. This connection, the exact course of which remains to be described, terminates in the lateral basal amygdaloid nucleus.

4b. WHITLOCK and NAUTA [180, 267] have found that the inferior temporal gyrus projects to the basolateral and central amygdaloid nuclei. According to HERZOG and VAN HOESEN [97] this projection originates from a much larger portion of the temporal cortex, which includes the rostral parts of the superior, the middle as well as the inferior temporal gyri.

4c. Apart from the temporal cortex, the orbitofrontal cortex has also been reported to send fibres to the amygdala [127, 256]. Following medial prefrontal ablations in rhesus monkeys, LEICHNITZ and ASTRUC [150] found degeneration in the basal, lateral and central amygdaloid nuclei. The degenerating fibres appeared to follow a peculiar course. Passing caudally, these fibres entered the stria terminalis; however, at midthalamic levels they left this bundle and descended through the internal capsule, the globus pallidus and the substantia innominata to the amygdaloid complex.

The efferent projections of the amygdaloid complex distribute to (1) the septopreopticohypothalamic continuum, (2) the dorsal thalamus, (3) the reticular formation and various other cell groups located in the brain stem and (4) a number of areas of the cerebral cortex (Figs. 143 and 144). These connections may be documented as follows:

1a. A large number of fibres originating mainly but not exclusively from the corticomedial nuclear group passes with the stria terminalis to the area directly dorsocaudal to the anterior commissure where they split up into the three components already mentioned. The fibres of the precommissural component curve caudally around the anterior commissure and terminate in the medial preoptic and anterior hypothalamic areas as well as in the ventromedial hypothalamic nucleus [61, 93, 159]. The fibres of the commissural component connect the two cortical amygdaloid nuclei [145]. The fibres of the postcommissural component spread to the bed nucleus of the stria terminalis, an elongated cell mass that accompanies the stria terminalis throughout most of its extent, and to the area of the anterior hypothalamic nucleus. These postcommissural fibres originate mainly from the medial, basal and lateral amygdaloid nuclei [151].

1b. Fibres originating from the basolateral nuclear group and from the cortical areas surrounding the amygdala have been reported to pass via the ventral amygdalofugal pathway to a variety of structures among which the medio-frontal cortex, the basal septal region and the lateral preopticohypothalamic zone may be mentioned [180, 183].

2. A certain proportion of the ventral amygda-lofugal fibres join the inferior thalamic peduncle and pass to the medial nucleus of the thalamus [130, 132, 180]. It is noteworthy that according to HEIMER [92] most of the ventral amygdalofu-gal fibres, described previously as projecting to the lateral preopticohypothalamic zone, do not terminate in this zone, but rather represent fibres of passage to the medial thalamic nu-cleus.

3. The nucleus centralis amygdalae gives rise to a projection that after having traversed the substantia innominata and the hypothalamus descends into the brain stem extending as far caudal as the obex level. The fibres of this so-called amygdalotegmental bundle supply the lateral hypothalamus, the ventral tegmental area, the periaqueductal grey, the mesencephal-ic and rhombencephalic parts of the reticular formation and the dorsal motor nucleus of the vagus [105a].

4. The investigations of KRETTEK and PRICE [130–133] have shown that in the rat and cat projections arising in specific amygdaloid nuclei terminate in distinct areas of the cerebral cortex. For details the original papers should be consulted. Suffice it to mention here that the cortical and basolateral nuclei send fibres to the entorhinal cortex and to the ventral subicu-lum [131, 133], whereas certain portions of the basolateral nucleus project to the frontal areae 25 and 32, to the temporal areae 35 and 36, and to part of the insular cortex [132]. Recently, LLAMAS et al. [155] have provided evi-dence suggesting that in the cat the entire fron-tal cortex including the motor and premotor areas receive a direct projection from the basal magnocellular amygdaloid nucleus. As regards primates, our knowledge of the amygdalocorti-cal projections is still limited. In the rhesus monkey NAUTA [180] found projections of the amygdala to the orbital region of the prefrontal cortex, to the rostral parts of the superior, mid-dle and inferior temporal gyri, as well as to the ventral insular area. JACOBSON and TROJA-NOWSKI [113] reported that in the same species the lateral division of the basal amygdaloid nucleus projects to the prefrontal granular cortex.

The *hippocampus* or *hippocampal formation* is a large C-shaped structure that forms part of the medial wall of the cerebral hemi-sphere. This structure can be subdivided morphologically into three parts, the hippo-campus praecommissuralis, the hippo-campus supracommissuralis and the hippo-campus retrocommissuralis (Fig. 23). The two parts first mentioned are relatively small, vestigial structures; the retrocommis-sural hippocampus, on the other hand, is well developed and represents the main por-tion of the hippocampal formation. The names of the three parts, it should be noted, refer to their position with respect to the corpus callosum. The precommissural hip-pocampus consists of a narrow, vertically oriented structure, situated in the caudal part of the area subcallosa just rostral to the septum verum (Fig. 136). This structure continues dorsorostrally into the indusium griseum, a strand of hippocampal tissue which extends the whole length of the corpus callosum. The indusium griseum represents the hippocampus supracommis-suralis. Two small fibre bundles, the medial and lateral longitudinal striae, are embed-ded in it (Fig. 23). These bundles represent a small supracallosal component of the for-nix. The principal subcallosal fornix will be discussed below. In the region of the splenium of the corpus callosum the hippo-campus supracommissuralis passes over into the hippocampus retrocommissuralis, the expanded, morphologically most caudal portion of the hippocampal formation. This structure, which is situated in the medial part of the temporal lobe, during ontogen-esis rolls in on itself along a longitudinal groove, the hippocampal sulcus. Due to this infolding the retrocommissural hippo-campus protrudes into the inferior horn of the lateral ventricle (Fig. 138). The most rostral portion of the retrocommissural hippocampus is recurved dorsally and constitutes a rounded swelling known as the uncus (Figs. 11, 23 and 136).

The hippocampal formation constitutes the archipallial part of the cerebral hemisphere; it contains a relatively simple three-layered allocortex throughout its extent. The retrocommissural hippocampus is clearly differentiated into three longitudinally arranged structures: the fascia dentata, the cornu ammonis and the subiculum. The fascia dentata — the name refers to the toothed or beaded appearance of its surface — constitutes the most medial strip of the pallium. It is laterally continuous with the cornu ammonis, which in its turn passes over into the subiculum. Due to the infolding of the hippocampus the fascia dentata is on the upper side and the subiculum, on the lower side of the hippocampal sulcus (Figs. 61 and 62). The fascia dentata contains a granule cell layer of small neurons, whereas large, pyramidal elements prevail in both the cornu ammonis and the subiculum. On the medial surface of the hemisphere the subicular cortex is contiguous with the juxtallocortex or mesocortex. The latter represents a type of cortex that is transitional between the hippocampal allocortex and the neocortex. This transitional cortex covers the parahippocampal gyrus and is also found in the supracallosal cingulate gyrus.

The cingulate gyrus, which borders on the vestigial precommissural and supracallosal parts of the hippocampus, is in the area behind the splenium of the corpus callosum directly continuous with the parahippocampal gyrus. The hippocampus, the parahippocampal gyrus and the cingulate gyrus constitute together a large arcuate convolution known as the limbic lobe (Fig. 4). The allocortical hippocampus forms the 'inner ring', whereas the mesocortical parahippocampal and cingulate gyri form the 'outer ring' of that lobe (Fig. 133).

Before focussing on the afferent and efferent connections of the hippocampus, two large limbic fibre bundles, viz. the cingulum and the fornix, should be briefly commented upon. The cingulum is a bundle of short and long association fibres which surrounds the corpus callosum. Passing through the core of the cingulate and parahippocampal gyri it extends from the septal area to the uncus region in the temporal lobe (Figs. 134 and 147). The fornix is a compact fibre bundle connecting the hippocampus with the hypothalamus and with various other structures (Figs. 23 and 138). Its fibres first form the alveus, a thin white layer on the ventricular surface of the cornu ammonis, and then converge as the fimbria along the medial aspect of the hippocampus. Running posterosuperiorly, the fibres of the fimbria enter the crus of the fornix, a flattened structure that arches upwards and medially under the splenium of the corpus callosum. In this region a number of fibres decussate to the opposite side, thus constituting the commissure of the fornix (Fig. 138). Proceeding rostrally over the thalamus, the two crura converge and join to form the corpus of the fornix, which lies immediately beneath the corpus callosum. However, at the level of the anterior pole of the thalamus the fornical corpus separates again into two bundles, the columns of the fornix, which curve ventrally in front of the interventricular foramen and caudal to the anterior commissure to enter the hypothalamus. Immediately behind the interventricular foramen a considerable number of fibres leave the column and pass backwards to the anterior nucleus of the thalamus and to the bed nucleus of the stria terminalis (Fig. 146). Other fibres split off from the fornix just above the anterior commissure and constitute a small precommissural portion of the fornix (Figs. 138 and 146). The main bundle of the fornix or postcommissural fornix finally traverses the hypothalamus, where most of its fibres terminate in the mamillary body (Figs. 134 and 136).

The hippocampus receives afferent fibres from (1) the area entorhinalis, (2) the septum, (3) the hypothalamus and (4) the rostral brainstem (Figs. 145, 152 and 154). These connections may be documented as follows:

1. The most conspicuous and quantitatively most important input to the hippocampus is formed by afferents from the area entorhinalis. These fibres terminate in the fascia dentata as well as in the cornu ammonis [100, 241]. The entorhinal area, in its turn, receives a large projection from the subiculum [228, 229] as well as from the cornu ammonis [99, 220] and is also in communication with other widespread areas of the cerebral cortex. Thus, it receives fibres from the prepiriform cortex, the frontal cortex and from the inferior part of the temporal cortex [258, 259, 260]. Fibres originating from the cingulate gyrus reach the entorhinal area by way of the cingulum. Subcortical afferents of the entorhinal area include (1) a large projection from the anterior thalamic nucleus which, like the cingulate fibres, passes through the cingulum [64, 65, 230] and (2) fibres from the amygdala [16, 131, 133]. It is noteworthy that a certain proportion of the cingulum fibres [2, 258] and the fibres arising from the amygdala [131, 133] bypass the entorhinal cortex and terminate directly in the subiculum.

2. The medial septal nucleus and the adjacent nucleus of the diagonal band of Broca send by way of the fornix fibres to the cornu ammonis and the subiculum [122, 167]; according to DOMESICK [66] the fibres from the nucleus of the diagonal band terminate also in the fascia dentata.

3. It has been recently reported that in the rat [271] and in the squirrel monkey [62] several hypothalamic areas, including the periventricular and lateral hypothalamic areas and the supramamillary nucleus project to the hippocampus.

4. In the rat [271] the hippocampus receives a direct input from the interpeduncular nucleus, the superior central nucleus, the dorsal raphe nucleus, the dorsal tegmental nucleus and the locus coeruleus. Several of these connections have been demonstrated to contain monoaminergic fibres [206, 208] (cf. Figs. 152 and 154).

A discussion of the complex intrinsic connections of the hippocampus falls outside the scope of the present work. Suffice it to mention that the axons of the dentate granule cells terminate in a highly ordered manner within the cornu ammonis [22] and that the latter sends fibres to the subiculum [101, 220] (Fig. 145). These connections presumably constitute a directionally polarized, sequential pathway, whereby input to the hippocampus passes successively through the fascia dentata and the cornu ammonis to the subiculum where, as has been recently established, the majority of all hippocampal efferents, both cortical and subcortical, originate [220].

Turning now to the efferent connections of the hippocampus, it should be stated first of all that investigations with the aid of the recently developed tracer techniques have brought a radical change in our insights concerning the organisation of these connections. Contrary to what has been believed for almost a century, the entire postcommissural fornix and a considerable part of the precommissural fornix originate from the subiculum rather than from the cornu ammonis. The contribution of the latter structure to the fornix has been shown to be only minor and to be confined to the precommissural fornix. In the light of these findings the hippocampal efferents may be grouped as follows: (1) efferents of the cornu ammonis, (2) contributions of the subiculum to the precommissural fornix, (3) contributions of the subiculum to the postcommissural fornix and (4) 'nonfornical' efferents.

This distribution of the fibres of these four groups is diagrammatically represented in Figure 146 and may be documented as follows:

1. The precommissural fornix fibres originating from the cornu ammonis terminate exclusively in the lateral part of the septum [240, 241].

2. The precommissural fornix fibres originating from the subiculum are distributed to the lateral septum, the medial parts of the nucleus accumbens, the anterior olfactory nucleus, the precommissural hippocampus, the medial part of the frontal cortex and to the gyrus rectus [220, 241].

3. The postcommissural fornix exclusively contains, apart from some hippocampal afferents, fibres originating from the subiculum. Most of these fibres terminate in the mamillary body; smaller contingents are distributed to the anterior thalamic nucleus, the bed nucleus of the stria terminalis and the area of the ventromedial hypothalamic nucleus [166, 220, 240, 241].

4. The subiculum projects to various cortical areas, including the entorhinal area and parts of the adjacent medial temporal cortex, the retrosplenial and caudal cingulate areas and the caudal part of the medial frontal cortex [220]. It is known that bilateral lesions of the hippocampus lead to a dramatic loss of recent memory. Lack of this disorder following bilateral fornix destruction may well be indicative of the relative importance of the direct subiculocortical efferents just mentioned [220]. In addition to these cortical efferents the subiculum sends fibres to the amygdala [220].

The postcommissural fornix forms part of a closed system of centres and connections in which both the inner and the outer ring of the limbic lobe are involved. This system, which has already been briefly discussed, is known as the circuit of Papez (Fig. 147). The structures constituting the outer ring, i.e., the cingulate and parahippocampal gyri, receive impulses from wide areas of the neocortex and convey these impulses by way of the cingulum towards the inner ring. Thus, it appears that the mesocortical outer ring not only positionally and structurally but also functionally represents a zone of transition between the neocortex and the allocortical, hippocampal inner ring.

The *central olfactory system* or *rhinencephalon* is entirely confined to the telencephalon and comprises bilaterally the olfactory bulb, the olfactory tract and the basal olfactory area (Fig. 9). The olfactory bulb represents the primary centre for the reception of olfactory impulses. It is a small, flattened, ovoid body that rests on the cribriform plate of the ethmoid bone. Arising from the posterior pole of the bulb the olfactory tract passes backwards over the basal surface of the frontal lobe to become attached to the hemisphere. At its site of attachment the olfactory tract bifurcates into medial and lateral olfactory striae. The initial parts of these striae border together with the diagonal band of Broca a territory known as the anterior perforated substance. The medial olfactory stria extends towards the subcallosal area on the medial surface of the frontal lobe; the lateral olfactory stria passes laterally and then bends sharply around the limen insulae to enter the rostromedial part of the temporal lobe (Fig. 139). A small intermediate olfactory stria continues the course of the olfactory tract for a short distance and then fans out in the anterior perforated substance (Fig. 139). The basal olfactory area is formed by those grisea which receive direct projections from the olfactory bulb and includes the anterior olfactory nucleus, the olfactory tubercle, the prepiriform cortex and the cortical nucleus of the amygdala [219, 253]. The anterior olfactory nucleus consists of some small groups of neurons located in the caudal part of the olfactory bulb, in the olfactory tract and in the rostral-most part of the olfactory trigone. The olfactory tubercle (so named because its homologue in macrosmatic mammals is marked by a prominent elevation) is represented by a thin sheet of grey matter, situated in the area of the anterior perforated substance. The prepiriform cortex can be divided into two parts, a medial part overlying the lateral olfactory stria as it travels laterally across the base of the frontal lobe and a lateral part extending from the limen insulae over a small anteromedial area of the temporal lobe. Caudally the prepiriform cortex is replaced by the superficial, cortical nucleus of the amygdala. Except for the anterior olfactory nucleus, all grisea that receive direct olfactory afferents exhibit a laminated structure [253].

The receptive elements of the olfactory apparatus are slender, bipolar cells found in a specialised area of the nasal mucosa. These elements are provided with extremely fine axonal processes that accumulating in small bundles penetrate the cribriform plate and enter the olfactory bulb. Within the olfactory bulb the primary olfactory fibres enter into synaptic contact with various types of cells, among which the large mitral cells are the most conspicuous. The axons of these elements pass backwards in the olfactory tract and are distributed to the secondary olfactory areas mentioned above (Fig. 148). Experimental studies have conclusively shown that the macroscopic elevation known as the medial olfactory stria does not receive any secondary olfactory fibres [92, 219, 253]. After having distributed fibres to the anterior olfactory nucleus and to the olfactory tubercle, the entire secondary olfactory projection enters the lateral olfactory stria. Following that stria, the fibres reach the prepiriform cortex and the cortical amygdaloid nucleus where they terminate.

The most important tertiary olfactory projections and the various routes along which the rhinencephalon may discharge impulses to the reticulomotor apparatus of the brain stem are diagrammatically represented in Figure 148. These pathways require the following comments:

1. In many textbooks [25, 37, 51] the precommissural septum is considered to be an important nodal area in the olfactory projection system. This centre is described as receiving secondary olfactory fibres via a medial olfactory tract and as discharging via the medial forebrain bundle and the stria medullaris-habenulointerpeduncular pathway to the hypothalamus and to the midbrain tegmentum. As mentioned above it has been established that a medial olfactory tract carrying secondary olfactory fibres does not exist; however, this does not exclude the possibility of multisynaptic connections between the olfactory bulb and the precommissural septum.

2. As regards the efferents of the olfactory tubercle and of the olfactory cortex, the following observations have been reported [210, 227]: (1) Both centres send large numbers of fibres to the diencephalon; (2) A large proportion of these fibres descend in the medial forebrain bundle and terminate in the lateral preopticohypothalamic zone; (3) Other fibres leave the medial forebrain bundle to enter the inferior thalamic peduncle and to terminate in the medial thalamic nucleus. It is noteworthy that HEIMER [91, 92] has recently challenged the existence of a substantial olfactory projection to the lateral preopticohypothalamic zone. According to his observations, the fibres that were supposed to terminate there are actually en route to the medial thalamic nucleus.

3. HEIMER [91, 92] also was unable to confirm that fibres originating from the olfactory tubercle and the olfactory cortex pass by way of the stria medullaris to the habenular nuclei and terminate there. He observed that the fibres of the 'olfactory' portion of the stria medullaris which pass through the habenular region are on their way to the medial thalamic nucleus and do not emit terminal branches to that region.

4. The amygdala and the hippocampus presumably represent relay centres in polysynaptic routes by which the rhinencephalon is connected with the hypothalamus and ultimately

with the tegmentum of the midbrain. The successive links in these pathways have already been discussed.

Recent studies [28, 60, 64, 238] have shown that centrifugal fibres, originating from many different regions pass directly to the olfactory bulb. These regions include the anterior olfactory nucleus bilaterally and on the ipsilateral side the olfactory tubercle, the prepiriform cortex, the nucleus of the diagonal band of Broca, the lateral hypothalamic area, the (noradrenergic) locus coeruleus and the (serotonergic) dorsal raphe nucleus.

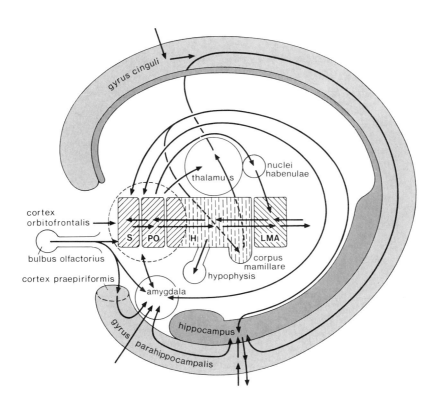

Fig. 133. Summary of the limbicohypothalamic complex. Subdivision of the area into central units and limbic rings, *H*, hypothalamus; *LMA*, limbic midbrain area; *PO*, preoptic region; *S*, septum

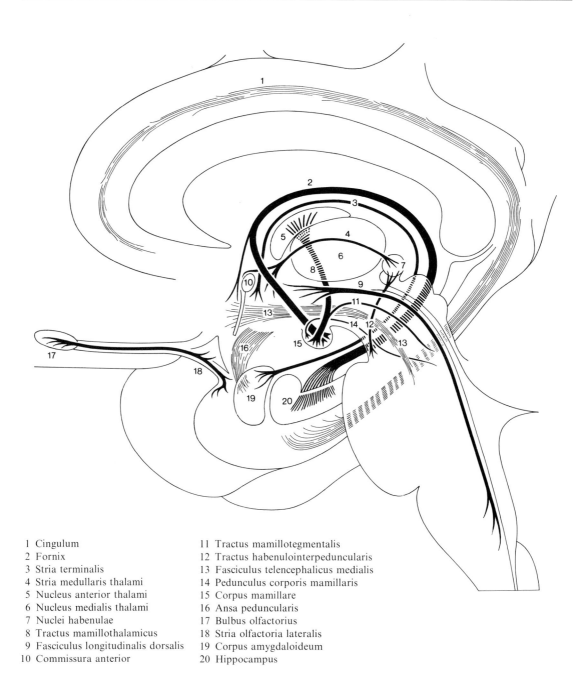

1 Cingulum
2 Fornix
3 Stria terminalis
4 Stria medullaris thalami
5 Nucleus anterior thalami
6 Nucleus medialis thalami
7 Nuclei habenulae
8 Tractus mamillothalamicus
9 Fasciculus longitudinalis dorsalis
10 Commissura anterior

11 Tractus mamillotegmentalis
12 Tractus habenulointerpeduncularis
13 Fasciculus telencephalicus medialis
14 Pedunculus corporis mamillaris
15 Corpus mamillare
16 Ansa peduncularis
17 Bulbus olfactorius
18 Stria olfactoria lateralis
19 Corpus amygdaloideum
20 Hippocampus

Fig. 134. The major pathways of the limbic system and the rhinencephalon

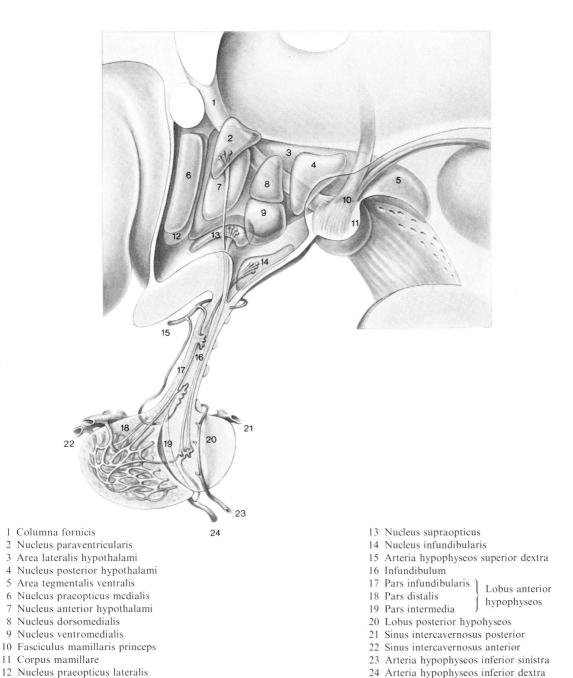

1 Columna fornicis
2 Nucleus paraventricularis
3 Area lateralis hypothalami
4 Nucleus posterior hypothalami
5 Area tegmentalis ventralis
6 Nuclcus praeopticus mcdialis
7 Nucleus anterior hypothalami
8 Nucleus dorsomedialis
9 Nucleus ventromedialis
10 Fasciculus mamillaris princeps
11 Corpus mamillare
12 Nucleus praeopticus lateralis

13 Nucleus supraopticus
14 Nucleus infundibularis
15 Arteria hypophyseos superior dextra
16 Infundibulum
17 Pars infundibularis ⎫
18 Pars distalis   ⎬ Lobus anterior hypophyseos
19 Pars intermedia   ⎭
20 Lobus posterior hypohyseos
21 Sinus intercavernosus posterior
22 Sinus intercavernosus anterior
23 Arteria hypophyseos inferior sinistra
24 Arteria hypophyseos inferior dextra

Fig. 135. The hypothalamic nuclei and the relationship between the hypothalamus and the pituitary gland (4/1 ×)

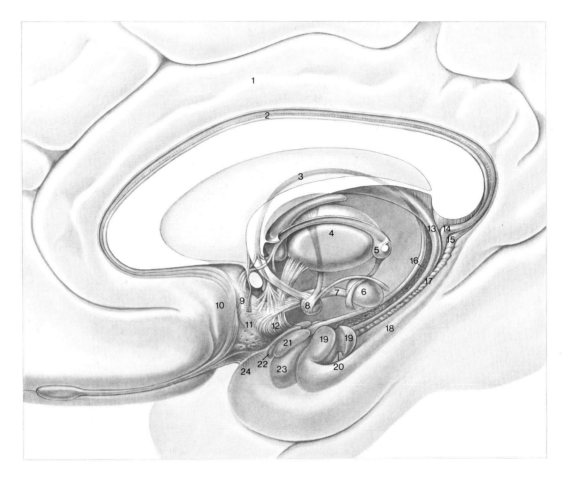

1 Gyrus cinguli
2 Indusium griseum
3 Stria terminalis
4 Nucleus medialis thalami
5 Nuclei habenulae
6 Nucleus ruber
7 Fasciculus telencephalicus medialis
8 Corpus mamillare
9 Septum verum
10 Area subcallosa
11 Gyrus diagonalis
12 Fibrae amygdalofugales ventrales

13 Crus fornicis
14 Gyrus fasciolaris
15 Fasciola cinerea
16 Fissura choroidea
17 Gyrus dentatus
18 Subiculum
19 Cornu ammonis
20 Site of limbus Giacomini
21 Nucleus corticalis amygdalae
22 Nucleus anterior amygdalae
23 Nuclei basalis + lateralis amygdalae
24 Cortex praepiriformis

Fig. 136. The structures of the limbic and olfactory systems and some input-output pathways as seen in a medial view ($3/2 \times$). Some displacement of structures serves to bring other structures in view. The walls of the third ventricle and the brain stem have been omitted almost completely; of the thalamus only the anterior, medial and habenular nuclei are illustrated

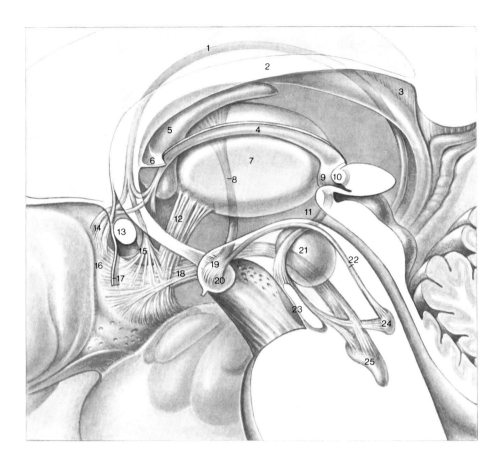

1 Stria terminalis
2 Fornix
3 Commissura fornicis
4 Stria medullaris thalami
5 Nucleus anterior thalami
6 Tela choroidea ventriculi tertii
7 Nucleus medialis thalami
8 Tractus mamillothalamicus
9 Nuclei habenulae
10 Commissura habenulae
11 Tractus habenulointerpeduncularis
12 Pedunculus thalami inferior
13 Commissura anterior

14 Precommissural { stria terminalis
    components of { stria medullaris thalami
                  { fornix
15 Stria terminalis postcommissuralis
16 Septum verum
17 Lamina terminalis
18 Fasciculus telencephalicus medialis
19 Fasciculus mamillaris princeps
20 Corpus mamillare
21 Nucleus ruber
22 Tractus mamillotegmentalis
23 Nucleus interpeduncularis
24 Nucleus tegmentalis dorsalis
25 Nucleus centralis superior

Fig. 137. The central part of the limbic area; medial view of nuclei and tracts (5/2 ×)

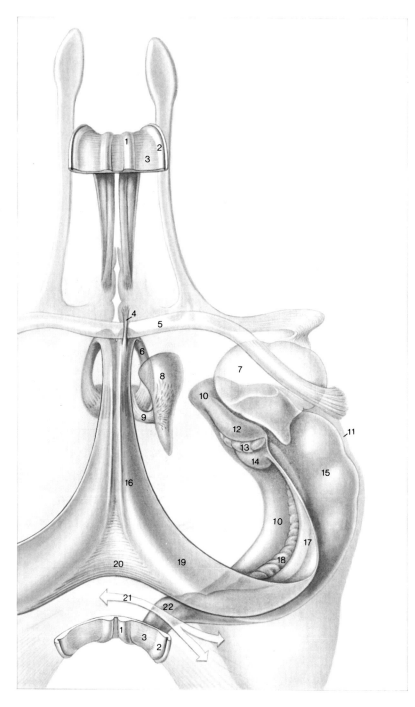

1 Stria longitudinalis medialis
2 Stria longitudinalis lateralis
3 Indusium griseum
4 Fornix praecommissuralis
5 Commissura anterior
6 Columna fornicis
7 Corpus amygdaloideum
8 Nucleus anterior thalami
9 Tractus mamillothalamicus
10 Subiculum
11 Ventriculus lateralis, cornu
    inferius
12 Cornu ammonis (gyrus
    uncinatus)
13 Limbus Giacomini
14 Cornu ammonis (gyrus
    intralimbicus)
15 Cornu ammonis (digitationes
    hippocampi)
16 Corpus fornicis
17 Fimbria hippocampi
18 Gyrus dentatus
19 Crus fornicis
20 Commissura fornicis
21 Site of corpus callosum
22 Gyrus fasciolaris

Fig. 138. The limbic structures isolated from most of their surroundings, seen from above (2/1 ×)

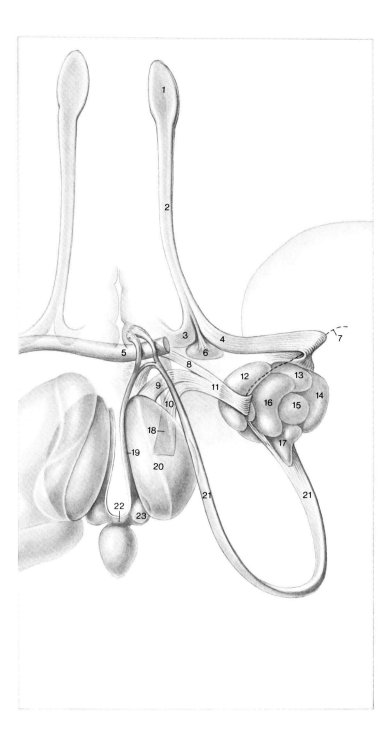

1 Bulbus olfactorius
2 Tractus olfactorius
3 Stria olfactoria medialis
4 Stria olfactoria lateralis
5 Commissura anterior
6 Tuberculum olfactorium
7 Limen insulae
8 Bandeletta diagonalis
9 Pedunculus thalami inferior
10 Fasciculus telencephalicus
   medialis
11 Fibrae amygdalofugales
   ventrales
12 Nucleus corticalis ⎫
13 Nucleus anterior   ⎪
14 Nucleus lateralis   ⎪ Corpus
15 Nucleus centralis   ⎬ amygdalo-
16 Nucleus medialis   ⎪ ideum
17 Nucleus basalis   ⎪
   (accessorius)   ⎭
18 Area lateralis hypothalami
19 Stria medullaris thalami
20 Nucleus medialis thalami
21 Stria terminalis
22 Commissura habenulae
23 Nuclei habenulae

Fig. 139. The rhinencephalic structures isolated from most of their surroundings, seen from above (2/1 ×). The *interrupted line* indicates the limen insulae and its continuation around the "hilus" of the temporal lobe

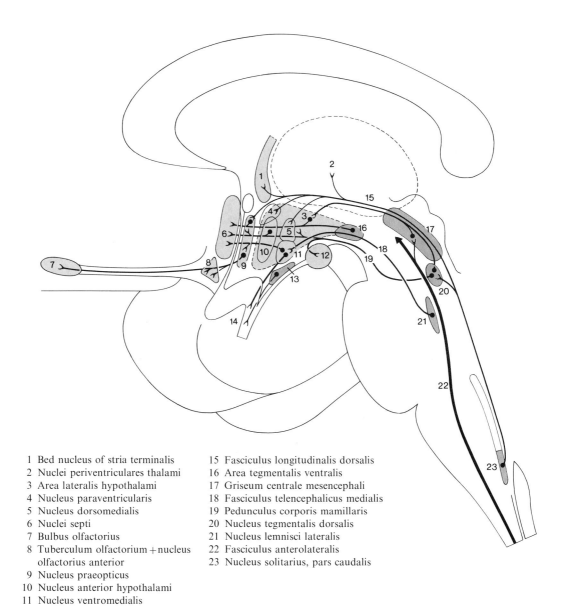

1 Bed nucleus of stria terminalis
2 Nuclei periventriculares thalami
3 Area lateralis hypothalami
4 Nucleus paraventricularis
5 Nucleus dorsomedialis
6 Nuclei septi
7 Bulbus olfactorius
8 Tuberculum olfactorium + nucleus
   olfactorius anterior
9 Nucleus praeopticus
10 Nucleus anterior hypothalami
11 Nucleus ventromedialis
12 Nucleus lateralis corporis mamillaris
13 Nucleus infundibularis
14 Infundibulum

15 Fasciculus longitudinalis dorsalis
16 Area tegmentalis ventralis
17 Griseum centrale mesencephali
18 Fasciculus telencephalicus medialis
19 Pedunculus corporis mamillaris
20 Nucleus tegmentalis dorsalis
21 Nucleus lemnisci lateralis
22 Fasciculus anterolateralis
23 Nucleus solitarius, pars caudalis

Fig. 140. Ascending connections of the basal prosencephalon

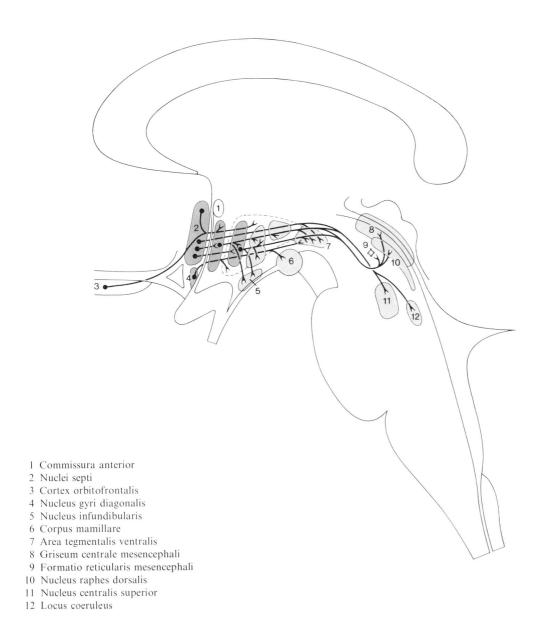

1 Commissura anterior
2 Nuclei septi
3 Cortex orbitofrontalis
4 Nucleus gyri diagonalis
5 Nucleus infundibularis
6 Corpus mamillare
7 Area tegmentalis ventralis
8 Griseum centrale mesencephali
9 Formatio reticularis mesencephali
10 Nucleus raphes dorsalis
11 Nucleus centralis superior
12 Locus coeruleus

Fig. 141 A. Descending connections of the basal prosencephalon; the medial forebrain bundle

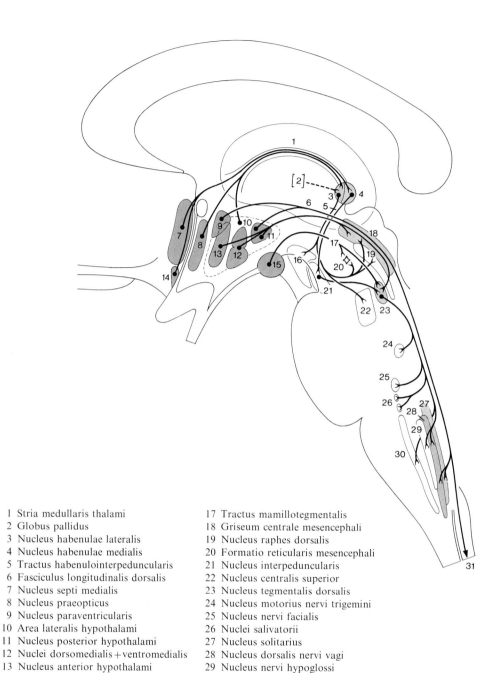

1 Stria medullaris thalami
2 Globus pallidus
3 Nucleus habenulae lateralis
4 Nucleus habenulae medialis
5 Tractus habenulointerpeduncularis
6 Fasciculus longitudinalis dorsalis
7 Nucleus septi medialis
8 Nucleus praeopticus
9 Nucleus paraventricularis
10 Area lateralis hypothalami
11 Nucleus posterior hypothalami
12 Nuclei dorsomedialis + ventromedialis
13 Nucleus anterior hypothalami
14 Nucleus gyri diagonalis
15 Corpus mamillare
16 Substantia nigra, pars compacta

17 Tractus mamillotegmentalis
18 Griseum centrale mesencephali
19 Nucleus raphes dorsalis
20 Formatio reticularis mesencephali
21 Nucleus interpeduncularis
22 Nucleus centralis superior
23 Nucleus tegmentalis dorsalis
24 Nucleus motorius nervi trigemini
25 Nucleus nervi facialis
26 Nuclei salivatorii
27 Nucleus solitarius
28 Nucleus dorsalis nervi vagi
29 Nucleus nervi hypoglossi
30 Nucleus ambiguus
31 Nucleus intermediolateralis (thoracic)

Fig. 141 B. Descending connections of the basal prosencephalon; descending tracts outside the medial forebrain bundle (dorsal tracts)

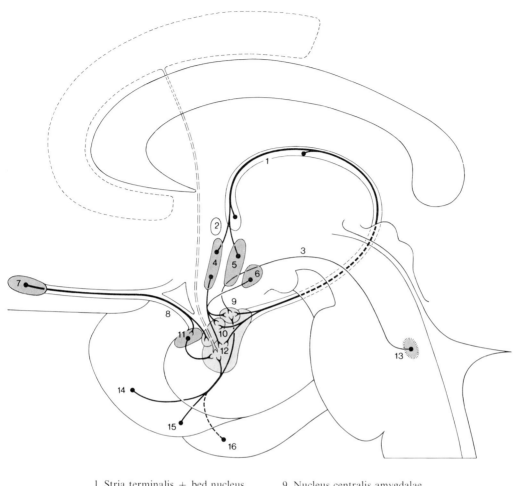

1 Stria terminalis + bed nucleus
2 Commissura anterior
3 Fasciculus telencephalicus medialis
4 Nucleus praeopticus
5 Nucleus anterior hypothalami
6 Nucleus ventromedialis
7 Bulbus olfactorius
8 Stria olfactoria lateralis

 9 Nucleus centralis amygdalae
10 Nuclei corticalis + medialis amygdalae
11 Cortex praepiriformis
12 Nuclei basalis + lateralis amygdalae
13 Nuclei parabrachiales
14 Gyrus temporalis superior ⎫ (cortex temporalis
15 Gyrus temporalis medius   ⎭   anterior)
16 Gyrus temporalis inferior (cortex temporalis lateralis)

Fig. 142. Afferent connections of the amygdaloid body

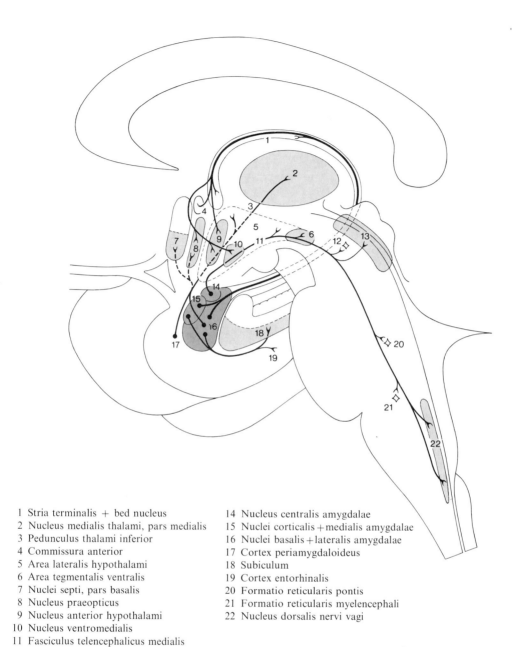

1 Stria terminalis + bed nucleus
2 Nucleus medialis thalami, pars medialis
3 Pedunculus thalami inferior
4 Commissura anterior
5 Area lateralis hypothalami
6 Area tegmentalis ventralis
7 Nuclei septi, pars basalis
8 Nucleus praeopticus
9 Nucleus anterior hypothalami
10 Nucleus ventromedialis
11 Fasciculus telencephalicus medialis
12 Formatio reticularis mesencephali
13 Griseum centrale mesencephali

14 Nucleus centralis amygdalae
15 Nuclei corticalis + medialis amygdalae
16 Nuclei basalis + lateralis amygdalae
17 Cortex periamygdaloideus
18 Subiculum
19 Cortex entorhinalis
20 Formatio reticularis pontis
21 Formatio reticularis myelencephali
22 Nucleus dorsalis nervi vagi

Fig. 143. Efferents of the amygdaloid body to the basal prosencephalon and the brain stem

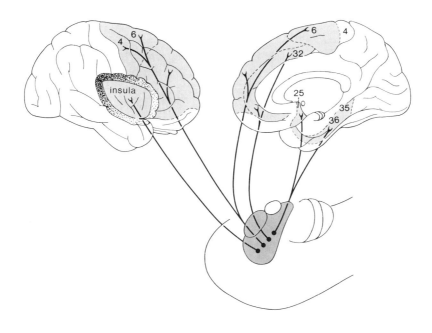

Fig. 144. Efferents of the amygdaloid body to the cerebral cortex. *Numbers* indicate fields of Brodmann (see Fig. 5)

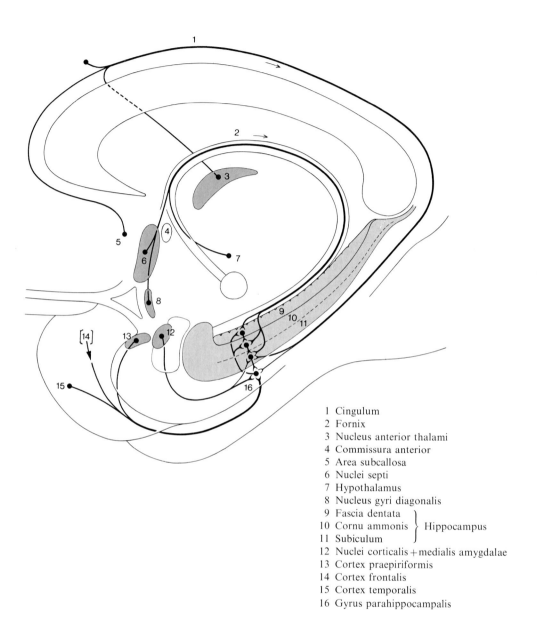

1 Cingulum
2 Fornix
3 Nucleus anterior thalami
4 Commissura anterior
5 Area subcallosa
6 Nuclei septi
7 Hypothalamus
8 Nucleus gyri diagonalis
9 Fascia dentata ⎫
10 Cornu ammonis ⎬ Hippocampus
11 Subiculum ⎭
12 Nuclei corticalis + medialis amygdalae
13 Cortex praepiriformis
14 Cortex frontalis
15 Cortex temporalis
16 Gyrus parahippocampalis

Fig. 145. Afferents of the hippocampus

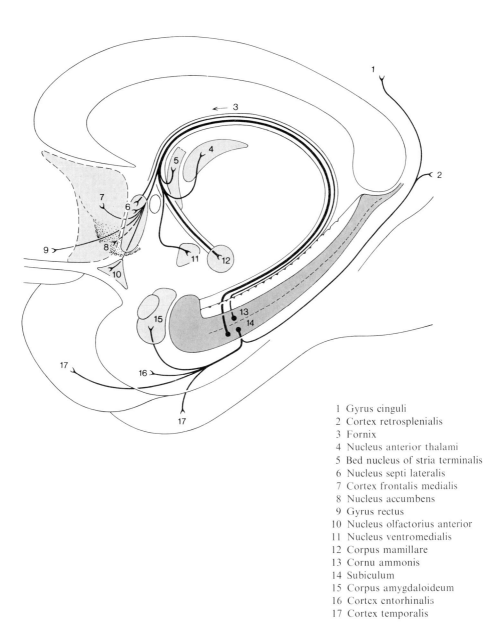

Fig. 146. Efferents of the hippocampus

1 Gyrus cinguli
2 Cortex retrosplenialis
3 Fornix
4 Nucleus anterior thalami
5 Bed nucleus of stria terminalis
6 Nucleus septi lateralis
7 Cortex frontalis medialis
8 Nucleus accumbens
9 Gyrus rectus
10 Nucleus olfactorius anterior
11 Nucleus ventromedialis
12 Corpus mamillare
13 Cornu ammonis
14 Subiculum
15 Corpus amygdaloideum
16 Cortex entorhinalis
17 Cortex temporalis

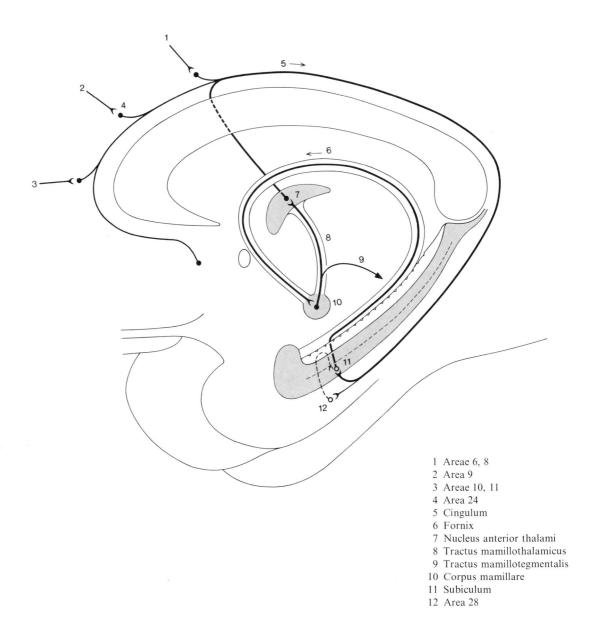

Fig. 147. The circuit of Papez

1 Areae 6, 8
2 Area 9
3 Areae 10, 11
4 Area 24
5 Cingulum
6 Fornix
7 Nucleus anterior thalami
8 Tractus mamillothalamicus
9 Tractus mamillotegmentalis
10 Corpus mamillare
11 Subiculum
12 Area 28

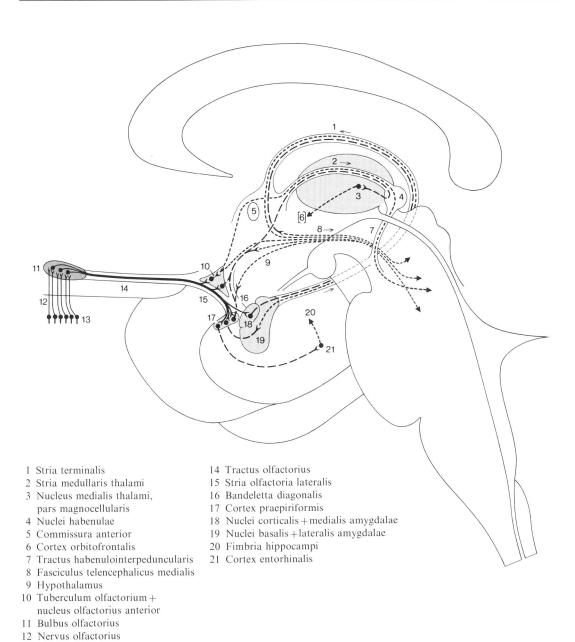

1 Stria terminalis
2 Stria medullaris thalami
3 Nucleus medialis thalami,
   pars magnocellularis
4 Nuclei habenulae
5 Commissura anterior
6 Cortex orbitofrontalis
7 Tractus habenulointerpeduncularis
8 Fasciculus telencephalicus medialis
9 Hypothalamus
10 Tuberculum olfactorium +
   nucleus olfactorius anterior
11 Bulbus olfactorius
12 Nervus olfactorius
13 Epithelium olfactorium

14 Tractus olfactorius
15 Stria olfactoria lateralis
16 Bandeletta diagonalis
17 Cortex praepiriformis
18 Nuclei corticalis + medialis amygdalae
19 Nuclei basalis + lateralis amygdalae
20 Fimbria hippocampi
21 Cortex entorhinalis

Fig. 148. The olfactory system. Primary, secondary and tertiary olfactory connections

Long Association and Commissural Connections

(Figs. 149 and 150)

Association fibres connect cortical areas within one hemisphere or between both hemispheres. Association fibres generally originate from supragranular layers, but terminate also in other layers of the neopallium [112, 119, 278].

Short association fibres may remain within the cortex or pass through the superficial white matter between neighbouring convolutions as U-fibres. Long association systems are located in deeper parts of the white matter, superficial to the corona radiata and the internal capsule. In the human brain long association systems are mainly known from gross dissection [59] and illustrated as such in Figure 150. Not much is known about their polarity, origin or termination. The following description is based on the experimental literature, which gives a fairly complete account of these connections in primates [118, 144, 199, 202, 261]. However, one should realise that the extent of the association cortex and the development of the association systems in the human brain far exceed those in experimental animals.

Short association fibres join the central convolutions with each other and the precentral gyrus with the premotor area (area 6) and also connect the postcentral gyrus with the rostral part of the superior and inferior parietal lobules (area 5). Long association fibres in the superior occipitofrontal fascicle connect parietal area 5 with frontal area 6 and more caudal parts of the parietal lobe (area 7) with the prefrontal cortex. The striate cortex (area 17) is connected with the peri-striate belt (area 18 and 19). The inferior longitudinal fascicle carries fibres that link the peristriate belt with the ventral part of the temporal lobe (area 20). The primary auditory cortex in the temporal operculum behaves in a similar fashion to the visual, the sensory and the motor cortex. Short fibres connect it with the neighbouring temporal cortex and this cortex gives rise to projections to more distant areas. Connections between the temporal and peristriate cortex and the inferior and superior parietal lobules constitute part of the anterior and posterior branches of the superior longitudinal fascicle. Reciprocal connections of the peristriate belt and the temporal lobe with the premotor area in the frontal lobe may use either the superior longitudinal fascicle or the inferior occipitofrontal fascicle. Both fascicles contribute to the capsula extrema and externa. The cortex of the temporal pole and the orbitofrontal cortex are linked by the uncinate fascicle, which runs in the limen insulae, through the ventral part of the claustrum and rostral to the anterior commissure. Widespread connections exist between the frontal, parietal and temporal cortex and the cingulate and parahippocampal convolutions. These fibres merge with other components to form the cingulum.

Fibres of the superior occipitofrontal fascicle are located medial to the corona radiata and ventral to the corpus callosum (Figs. 59 and 150). The bundle becomes less distinct caudally. Its origin and distribution is not known.

Commissural connections (Fig. 149) include the corpus callosum and the anterior commissure. The rostrum and genu of the corpus callosum fold around the anterior horn of the lateral ventricle. The truncus constitutes the roof of the central part of the lateral ventricle and fibres of the splenium spread out as the tapetum, which covers the roof and the lateral wall of the inferior and posterior horn. Most commissural connections are homotopical. Heterotopical connections terminate in the same areas in the contralateral hemisphere as those which receive association fibres on the ipsilateral side [199]. Orbitofrontal fibres occupy the rostrum, prefrontal fibres, the genu of the corpus callosum. Pericentral, parietal and temporal fibres are located in the truncus in that order. Occipital fibres are located in the splenium. Occipital fibres mainly originate from the peristriate belt region, whereas callosal connections of the striate region are limited to areas representing the middle of the visual field [199, 200, 204]. Both in the motor and the sensory cortex commissural fibres connect axial and girdle representation areas, but no commissural fibres arise or terminate in the hand and foot areas [204]. Few commissural fibres arise from the auditory cortex [199]. Commissural connections of the rostral one-third of the temporal lobe pass through the anterior commissure, together with the commissural portion of the stria terminalis and the commissural connections between the olfactory bulbs [201].

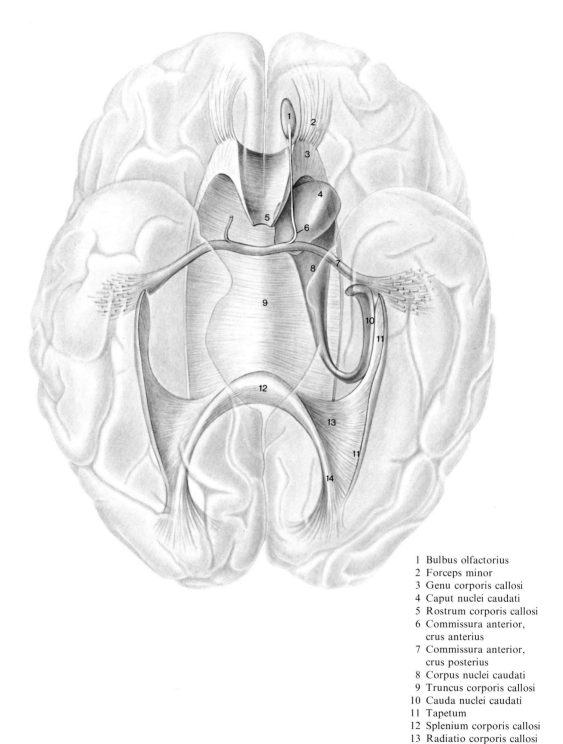

1 Bulbus olfactorius
2 Forceps minor
3 Genu corporis callosi
4 Caput nuclei caudati
5 Rostrum corporis callosi
6 Commissura anterior,
   crus anterius
7 Commissura anterior,
   crus posterius
8 Corpus nuclei caudati
9 Truncus corporis callosi
10 Cauda nuclei caudati
11 Tapetum
12 Splenium corporis callosi
13 Radiatio corporis callosi
14 Forceps major

Fig. 149. Commissural connections of the telencephalon as seen from the basal side of the brain(1/1×)

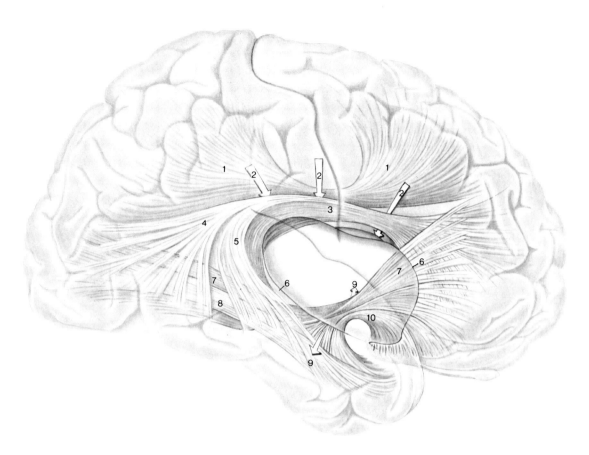

1 Fasciculus occipitofrontalis superior
2 Site of corona radiata
3 Fasciculus longitudinalis superior
4 Fasciculus longitudinalis superior, brachium posterius
5 Fasciculus longitudinalis superior, brachium anterius
6 Outline of insula
7 Fasciculus occipitofrontalis inferior
8 Fasciculus longitudinalis inferior
9 Site of commissura anterior
10 Fasciculus uncinatus

Fig. 150. Long association bundles of the right cerebral hemisphere in a lateral view (1/1×)

Monoamine Neuron Systems

The biogenic amines include the catecholamines, dopamine and noradrenaline, and the indoleamine, serotonin or 5-hydroxytryptamine. All three of these monoamines have a claim to be considered central neurotransmitters. Investigations carried out during the last 15 years have shown that a number of neuron groups, mainly situated in the brain stem, synthesise these monoamines and distribute them by fine-fibred, profusely ramifying projections to a great many regions of the brain and spinal cord. Although the mapping of these dopaminergic, noradrenergic and serotonergic neuron systems is still in full progress it seems appropriate to include some of the results obtained so far.

In the brain of the rat 15 catecholaminergic and 9 serotonergic cell groups have been identified [21, 55, 56, 85]. These cell groups have been designated as A1–A15 and B1–B9, respectively. This nomenclature will be followed as much as possible.

Dopaminergic Cell Groups and Pathways (Fig. 151)

Neurons which synthesise dopamine are found in the mesencephalon, the diencephalon and the telencephalon. The mesencephalic dopaminergic cells have been described as forming three cell groups, A8, A9 and A10, but the boundaries between these groups are indistinct [70, 109]. The cells of the A8 group are located in the mesencephalic reticular formation. This group merges ventromedially with the A9 group, which is constituted by the compact part of the substantia nigra. All of the cells present in the latter area have been reported to be monoaminergic [75]. The A10 group is an unpaired midline group that is limited ventrally by the interpeduncular nucleus. The majority of its cells are located within the confines of the ventral tegmental area. Four different dopaminergic cell groups, A11, A12, A13 and A14, have been recognized in the diencephalon [21, 70]. Group A11 is situated in the caudal hypothalamic periventricular region, dorsal to the infundibular nucleus, which contains most of the cells of the A12 group. The cells of the A13 group are located in the zona incerta, whereas those of the A14 group constitute a rostral continuation of the A12 group. As fas as is known the olfactory bulb is the only telencephalic centre containing dopaminergic neurons. These elements are scattered in the outer zone of the bulb and form part of a set of interneurons ('periglomerular cells'). They have been collectively designated the A15 group [85].

The cells of the A8 and A9 groups give rise to a large pathway that ascends in the lateral hypothalamic area from where its fibres successively diverge dorsally and laterally. After having traversed the internal capsule, these fibres fan out in the caudate nucleus and the putamen where they form a dense network of terminals. This *nigrostriatal dopaminergic system* [4, 254] is integrated into what has been called the third 'accessory' striatal circuit (Fig. 130). Some of the fibres of this system enter the central amygdaloid nucleus.

A second system, the *mesolimbic dopaminergic system*, originates mainly from the cells of the A10 group. Its fibres ascend medial to the nigrostriatal system in the medial forebrain bundle and are distributed to the following telencephalic structures: the bed nucleus of the stria terminalis, the olfactory tubercle, the nucleus accumbens [254], the lateral septal nucleus [152, 171], and certain parts of the frontal, cingulate and entorhinal cortex [153]. The cortical dopamine fibres in the areas mentioned constitute dense and well-delineated fields of termination.

A third dopaminergic system, which has been termed the *tubero-infundibular dopaminergic system*, arises from the cells of the A12 group. The axons of these cells pass to the rostroventral part of the infundibulum and innervate the external layer of the median eminence [254].

The cells of the groups A11, A13 and A14 finally give rise to a system of short, intradiencephalic projections which has been designated the *incerto-hypothalamic dopaminergic system* [20].

Noradrenergic Cell Groups and Pathways (Figs. 152 and 153)

Neurons that synthesise noradrenaline are restricted to the pontine and medullary tegmental regions. Seven noradrenergic cell groups, designated as A1–A7, have been described in rodents [55]. Most of these have also been recognised in primates [70, 75, 108, 188]. Groups A1 and A2 are both situated in the lower part of the medulla oblongata. The cells of group A1 surround the nucleus of the lateral funiculus and ex-

tend dorsomedially into the lateral part of the reticular formation; those of group A2 lie dorsal and lateral of the hypoglossal nucleus, close to the ventricular surface. Cells corresponding to group A3 in the rat, lying just dorsal to the inferior olivary complex, have not been observed in primates. Group A4 consists of a band of subependymal neurons which extends along the superior cerebellar peduncle. This group merges rostrally with the caudal portion of group A6. Group A5 consists of rather loosely arranged cells that surround the facial nucleus and the superior olivary complex. Group A6 is a densely packed accumulation of cells situated within the locus coeruleus. The latter is a macroscopically visible blue-black streak of tissue situated in the floor of the fourth ventricle at rostral pontine levels (Figs. 47, 68 and 69). Evidence suggests that all of the neurons situated in the central part of this structure are noradrenergic [75, 237]. The cells of group A7 are situated in the rostral pontine part of the lateral reticular formation. Strands of cells connect this cell group with the groups A4 and A6. Some authors [107] consider the groups A4, A6 and A7 together one complex.

The noradrenergic cell groups just discussed give rise to highly branched ascending and descending fibre systems that course the length of the neuraxis and form terminal networks in a variety of grisea. At present we have a fairly complete picture of the total distribution of noradrenergic fibres and terminal fields, but the extent to which individual terminal fields arise from separate neuronal groups is still a matter of dispute. In the present condensed and simplified survey a sharp and perhaps too sharp a distinction has been made between the projections of the locus coeruleus and those of the remaining noradrenergic cell groups. It is noteworthy that many of the noradrenergic fibre terminals are intimately associated with cerebral arterioles and capillaries. This relation suggests that the central noradrenergic system is involved in the regulation of cerebral blood flow [88, 89, 211, 239].

Containing almost half of the total number of noradrenaline synthesising neurons [242], the locus coeruleus is quantitatively by far the most important noradrenergic centre of the brain. Its efferents constitute a major ascending pathway designated the dorsal noradrenergic bundle [254]. Other efferents are distributed to the cerebellum and still others descend to the lower medulla oblongata and to the spinal cord (Fig. 152).

The *dorsal noradrenergic bundle* traverses the midbrain tegmentum in a position ventrolateral to the periaqueductal grey and then enters the hypothalamus, through the lateral part of which it proceeds to the septal region. From here the bundle ascends to enter the cingulum with which it encircles the corpus callosum. Along the course of the dorsal noradrenergic bundle distinct branches emerge to innervate a large number of mesencephalic, diencephalic and telencephalic grisea. The mesencephalic areas of termination include the central grey substance, the dorsal raphe nucleus and the superior and inferior colliculi. In the diencephalon branches following several different routes give rise to extensive terminal systems in many thalamic areas, most notably the anterior, ventral and lateral nuclear complexes and the medial and lateral geniculate bodies [154]. One branch follows the stria medullaris and supplies, apart from several thalamic centres, the medial and lateral habenular nuclei. As regards the hypothalamus, this region is generally believed to receive its noradrenergic innervation from the ventral

noradrenergic bundle (see below). Some authors [111, 115], however, have presented evidence suggesting that the hypothalamus is also supplied by fibres originating from the locus coeruleus. The main telencephalic areas of termination of the dorsal noradrenergic bundle and its branches are the amygdala (central, basal and lateral nuclei), the substantia innominata, the hippocampus (cornu ammonis and subiculum), the cingulate, retrosplenial and entorhinal cortical areas and the entire neocortex. The fibres to the amygdala and the adjacent cortical areas follow the course of the ventral amygdalofugal pathway; those to the hippocampus travel with the cingulum [242]. The fibres to the neocortex follow different courses. A large proportion traverses the internal and external capsules and the lentiform nucleus, others diverge from the cingulum, and still others pass forwards through the septal region [247]. It is important to note that the noradrenergic innervation of the neocortex is diffuse and uniform throughout [78, 254] and as such stands in sharp contrast to the dense and well-delineated cortical projections of the dopaminergic system.

The fibres passing from the locus coeruleus to the cerebellum follow the superior cerebellar peduncle and terminate in the central nuclei as well as in the cortex. The descending efferents of the locus coeruleus, supplemented by some fibres from the subcoeruleal A7 group, supply the dorsal nucleus of the vagus and certain parts of the inferior olivary complex and then constitute a massive pathway extending throughout the length of the cord. This ventrolateral coeruleospinal pathway gives rise to almost all noradrenergic terminals in the ventral horn and in the basal part of the dorsal horn [193].

From the foregoing survey of the efferents of the locus coeruleus this small centre appears to give rise to noradrenergic terminal fields in widely different areas of the brain and spinal cord. There is moreover evidence suggesting that single locus coeruleus neurons distribute collateral branches to the neocortex, the hippocampus, the cerebellum and the spinal cord [193, 194, 247, 254].

According to Ungerstedt [254] the cell groups A1, A2, A5 and A7 give rise to an ascending fibre system, which he termed the *ventral noradrenergic pathway*. This pathway ascends through the reticular core of the brain stem and continues rostrally mainly within the medial forebrain bundle. The terminal areas of this bundle include: in the mesencephalon, the ventrolateral part of the substantia grisea centralis and the reticular formation, in the diencephalon, the entire hypothalamus, especially the dorsomedial, periventricular, infundibular, supraoptic and paraventricular nuclei and the internal layer of the median eminence, and in the telencephalon, the preoptic area and the bed nucleus of the stria terminalis. Swanson and Hartman [242] confirmed the presence of noradrenergic terminals in all of these areas and described in addition a noradrenergic innervation of the olfactory bulb. However, these authors were unable to confirm the existence of a separate ventral noradrenergic pathway.

The cell groups A1, A2, A5 and A7 do not only project to higher levels of the brain, but have also been reported to give rise to descending bulbospinal fibres [56, 224, 254]. According to Dahlström and Fuxe [56], these fibres constitute two bulbospinal noradrenergic systems, one that descends mainly in the anterior funiculus and terminates in the ventral horn and another that descends in the dorsal part of the lateral funiculus and terminates in the intermediolateral nucleus and in the substantia gelatinosa.

Finally it may be mentioned that the dorsal vagus and the solitary nuclei receive a noradrenergic innervation, which, according to Ungerstedt [254], arises mainly from the A1 but, according to Swanson and Hartman [242], mainly from the A2 group.

Serotonergic Cell Groups and Pathways (Fig. 154)

Serotonin-containing neurons occur in the mesencephalon, pons and medulla oblongata, but in all of these parts of the brain the elements mentioned are essentially confined to the median and paramedian zones. In marked contrast to most of the catecholaminergic cell groups, the serotonergic neurons are mainly distributed within specific cytoarchitectonic entities, namely the nuclei of the raphe. Dahlström and Fuxe [55, 56] described nine groups of serotonergic cells (B1–B9) in the brain stem of the rat. Most of these have also been recognised in primates [70, 109]. In the following synopsis the nomenclature of Dahlström and Fuxe will be employed. The description of the various raphe nuclei follows, as much as possible, those of Taber et al. [244] and Braak [27].

Cell group B1 is situated in the ventral part of the medulla oblongata and borders ventrally on the pyramidal tracts. It is limited mainly to the nucleus raphes pallidus, although some of its cells extend laterally in the ventral part of the reticular formation. The rostral part of group B1 is continuous with the caudal part of group B3. Cell group B2 is situated at the same level as group B1, but occupies a more dorsal position. Its cells form two narrow paramedian sheets that coincide with the nucleus raphes obscurus. Cell group B3 is situated in the borderland between the medulla oblongata and the pons. Most of its cells are found within the nucleus raphes magnus, but others constitute laterally extending bands along the fibre bundles of the corpus trapezoideum. Group B5 is rather small and located within the nucleus raphes pontis at the level of the motor nucleus of the fifth nerve. In the upper pons and lower midbrain the data derived from cytoarchitectonic studies are difficult to reconcile with those resulting from histofluorescence studies on the distribution of serotonergic cells. However, it seems likely that the cell groups B6 and B8 both lie largely within the confines of the superior central nucleus of Bechterew. This nucleus is situated in the upper part of the tegmentum pontis and extends rostrally into the tegmentum of the midbrain. The large, mesencephalic cell group B7 is mainly localised within the nucleus dorsalis raphes. The latter is situated in and ventral to the periaqueductal grey. It extends from the level of the dorsal tegmental nucleus to the caudal pole of the oculomotor nucleus. The ventral part of the nucleus is situated between the two medial longitudinal fascicles. It has been recently reported [44] that in the rat several diencephalic centres, including the dorsomedial and ventromedial hypothalamic nuclei and the habenular and mamillary nuclei also contain indoleamine neurons.

With regard to its fibre projections, the serotonin-containing neuronal system shares several characteristics with the central noradrenergic system. Both systems give rise to ascending and descending axons and both distribute fibres to the cerebral as well as to the cerebellar cortex. In Figure 154 some of the serotonergic pathways are schematically represented. It should be emphasised that the data derived from studies with fluorescence histochemical techniques [55, 56, 74, 254] are supplemented with the results of analyses of the efferent connections of the raphe nuclei with anterograde [23, 46, 245] and retrograde [207, 221] tracer techniques. Since all of the raphe nuclei contain a certain proportion of non-serotonergic cells, it may well be that some of the projections depicted are in fact non-serotonergic.

The fibre systems represented in Figure 154 can be designated as follows: (1) the ventral ascending pathway, (2) the dorsal ascending pathway, (3) the cerebellar pathway, (4) the descending propriobulbar pathway, and (5) bulbospinal pathways. These pathways may be documented as follows: 1. The large *ventral ascending serotonergic pathway* arises mainly from the cell groups B6–B8. Its fibres sweep ventrally from these nuclei and then curve rostrally to course through the ventral tegmentum into the lateral hypothalamic area. During its course through the midbrain, fibres are given off to the interpeduncular nucleus and to the substantia nigra [23, 198, 245]. Other fibres ascend in the habenulointerpeduncular tract and terminate in the habenular nuclei and in various thalamic centres including the medial, parafascicular and midline nuclei [23, 46]. The bundle distributes fibres along its diencephalic course to the lateral hypothalamic area [23, 245], the mamillary body, the caudate nucleus and the putamen [23, 74] and to the neocortex. The latter pass laterally through the internal and external capsules. In front of the hypothalamus the ventral ascending serotonergic pathway splits up into fibre groups of varying size: (a) Some fibres proceed rostrally to terminate in the preoptic region, the septum, the olfactory tubercle, the olfactory bulb and the frontal neocortex. (b) Other fibres arch laterally and pass via the ansa peduncularis to the nucleus of the diagonal band of Broca, to the amygdala [266] and to the prepiriform and anterior entorhinal cortex [23]. (c) Still other fibres supply the accumbens nucleus and the anterior parts of the caudate nucleus and the putamen. (d) Finally, a conspicuous bundle ascends dorsally into the cingulum to reach, eventually, the hippocampus via a caudal approach. During its course fibres are given off to the cingulate and entorhinal cortex. In the hippocampus the cingulate projection sprays out into the subiculum and the cornu ammonis [23, 172].

2. The *dorsal ascending serotonergic pathway* is formed by fibres that emerge from the cell groups B3, B5 and B7. These fibres pass rostrally along with the periventricular dorsal longitudinal fascicle of SCHÜTZ and terminate in the mesencephalic central grey and in the posterior hypothalamic area [23].

3. The *cerebellar serotonergic pathway* emerges mainly from the cell groups B5 and B6 and passes with the pedunculus cerebellaris medius to the cerebellum where its fibres are distributed to both the cortex and the deep nuclei [23].

4. The *descending propriobulbar serotonergic pathway* consists of fibres that pass from the cell groups B6–B8 and B3 and B5 to lower levels of the brain stem. The dorsal raphe and superior central nuclei send fibres to the dorsal tegmental nucleus, the locus coeruleus and the pontine and medullary reticular formation [23, 46, 221, 245]. The more caudally situated nucleus raphes pontis and nucleus raphes magnus project likewise to the reticular formation and the cell mass last mentioned sends in addition fibres to the inferior olivary complex [23].

5. The *bulbospinal serotonergic projections* are formed by fibres that arise from cell groups B1–B3. In the spinal cord most of these fibres descend in the anterior funiculus and in the anterior part of the lateral funiculus to innervate the ventral horn. The remaining fibres descend in the dorsal part of the lateral funiculus to innervate the dorsal horn and the autonomic intermediolateral nucleus [254].

From the foregoing survey it appears that the serotonergic system sends most of its efferents to limbic structures and to the reticular formation. It is also remarkable that the principal noradrenergic cell mass, i.e., the locus coeruleus, receives its most important afferent projection from the nucleus raphes dorsalis, the largest serotonergic centre [221].

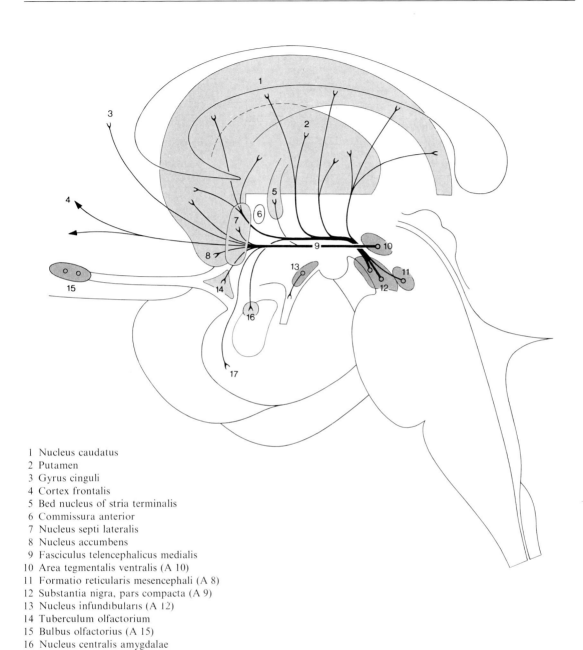

1 Nucleus caudatus
2 Putamen
3 Gyrus cinguli
4 Cortex frontalis
5 Bed nucleus of stria terminalis
6 Commissura anterior
7 Nucleus septi lateralis
8 Nucleus accumbens
9 Fasciculus telencephalicus medialis
10 Area tegmentalis ventralis (A 10)
11 Formatio reticularis mesencephali (A 8)
12 Substantia nigra, pars compacta (A 9)
13 Nucleus infundibularis (A 12)
14 Tuberculum olfactorium
15 Bulbus olfactorius (A 15)
16 Nucleus centralis amygdalae
17 Cortex entorhinalis

Fig. 151. The dopaminergic system

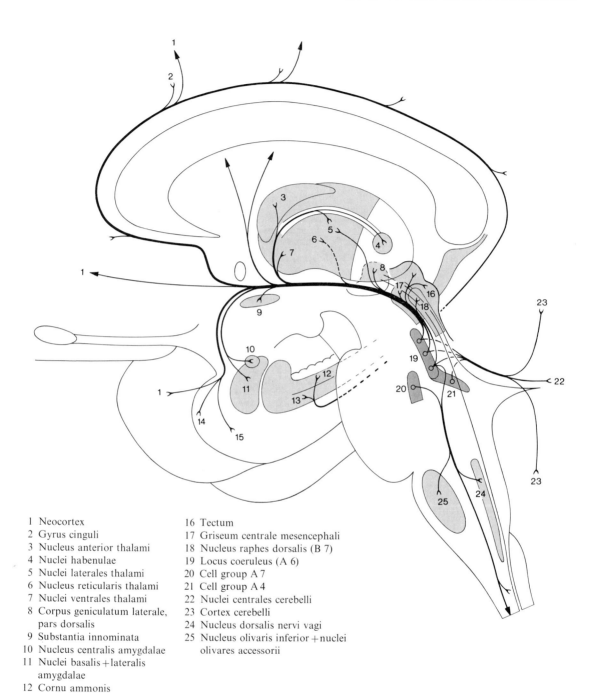

1 Neocortex
2 Gyrus cinguli
3 Nucleus anterior thalami
4 Nuclei habenulae
5 Nuclei laterales thalami
6 Nucleus reticularis thalami
7 Nuclei ventrales thalami
8 Corpus geniculatum laterale,
   pars dorsalis
9 Substantia innominata
10 Nucleus centralis amygdalae
11 Nuclei basalis + lateralis
   amygdalae
12 Cornu ammonis
13 Subiculum
14 Cortex piriformis
15 Cortex entorhinalis

16 Tectum
17 Griseum centrale mesencephali
18 Nucleus raphes dorsalis (B 7)
19 Locus coeruleus (A 6)
20 Cell group A 7
21 Cell group A 4
22 Nuclei centrales cerebelli
23 Cortex cerebelli
24 Nucleus dorsalis nervi vagi
25 Nucleus olivaris inferior + nuclei
   olivares accessorii

Fig. 152. The noradrenergic system I: connections of the locus coeruleus

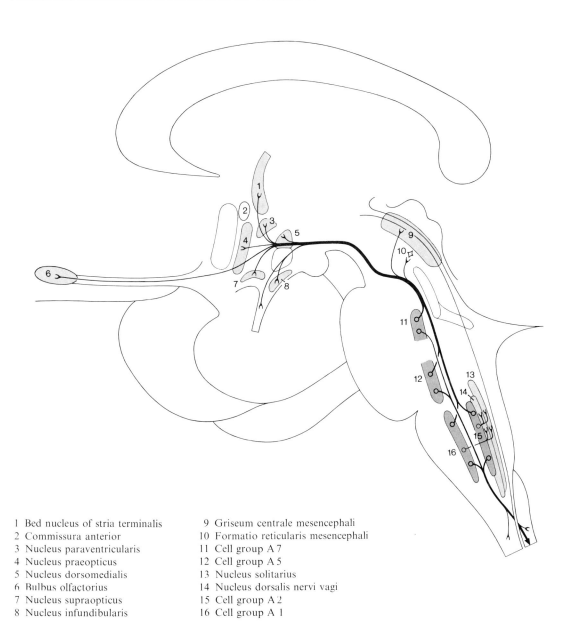

1 Bed nucleus of stria terminalis
2 Commissura anterior
3 Nucleus paraventricularis
4 Nucleus praeopticus
5 Nucleus dorsomedialis
6 Bulbus olfactorius
7 Nucleus supraopticus
8 Nucleus infundibularis

9 Griseum centrale mesencephali
10 Formatio reticularis mesencephali
11 Cell group A 7
12 Cell group A 5
13 Nucleus solitarius
14 Nucleus dorsalis nervi vagi
15 Cell group A 2
16 Cell group A 1

Fig. 153. The noradrenergic system II: connections of other cell groups

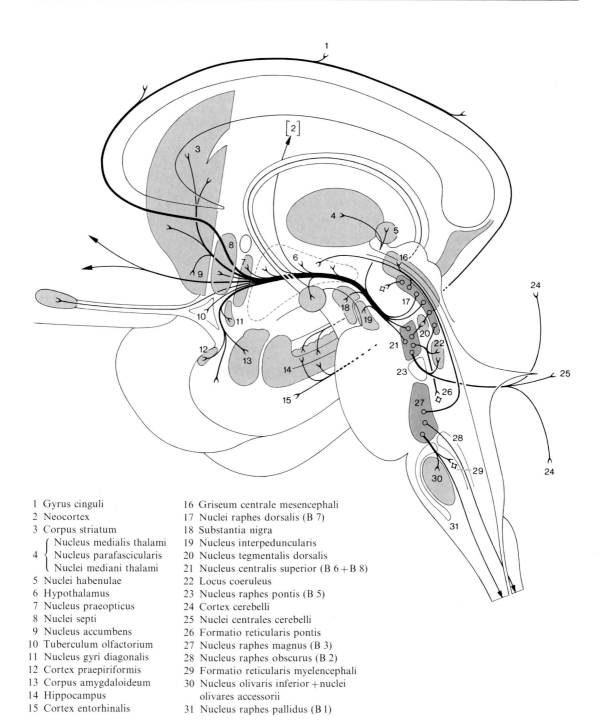

1 Gyrus cinguli
2 Neocortex
3 Corpus striatum
4 ⎧ Nucleus medialis thalami
   ⎨ Nucleus parafascicularis
   ⎩ Nuclei mediani thalami
5 Nuclei habenulae
6 Hypothalamus
7 Nucleus praeopticus
8 Nuclei septi
9 Nucleus accumbens
10 Tuberculum olfactorium
11 Nucleus gyri diagonalis
12 Cortex praepiriformis
13 Corpus amygdaloideum
14 Hippocampus
15 Cortex entorhinalis

16 Griseum centrale mesencephali
17 Nuclei raphes dorsalis (B 7)
18 Substantia nigra
19 Nucleus interpeduncularis
20 Nucleus tegmentalis dorsalis
21 Nucleus centralis superior (B 6 + B 8)
22 Locus coeruleus
23 Nucleus raphes pontis (B 5)
24 Cortex cerebelli
25 Nuclei centrales cerebelli
26 Formatio reticularis pontis
27 Nucleus raphes magnus (B 3)
28 Nucleus raphes obscurus (B 2)
29 Formatio reticularis myelencephali
30 Nucleus olivaris inferior + nuclei
   olivares accessorii
31 Nucleus raphes pallidus (B 1)

Fig. 154. The serotonergic system

References

1. Aghajanian, G.K., Wang, R.Y.: Habenular and other midbrain raphe afferents demonstrated by a modified retrograde tracing technique. Brain Res. *122*, 229–242 (1977)

2. Alksne, J.F., Blackstad, T.W., Walberg, F., White L.E. (Jr.): Electron microscopy of axon degeneration: A valuable tool in experimental neuroanatomy. Ergebn. Anat. Entwicklungsgesch. *39*, 1–32 (1966)

3. Altman, J., Carpenter, M.B.: Fiber projections of the superior colliculus in the cat. J. Comp. Neurol. *116*, 157–178 (1961)

4. Andén, N.E., Carlsson, A., Dahlström, A., Fuxe, K., Hillarp, N.A., Larsson, K.: Demonstration and mapping out of nigroneostriatal dopamine neurons. Life Sci. *3*, 523–530 (1964)

5. Andén, N.E., Dahlström, A., Fuxe, K., Larsson, K., Olson, L., Ungerstedt, U.: Ascending monoamine neurons to the telencephalon and diencephalon. Acta Physiol. Scand. *67*, 313–326 (1966)

6. Andy, O.J., Stephan, H.: The septum in the human brain. J. Comp. Neurol. *133*, 383–410 (1968)

7. Angaut, P., Brodal, A.: The projection of the "vestibulocerebellum" onto the vestibular nuclei in the cat. Arch. Ital. Biol. *105*, 441–479 (1967)

8. Angevine J.B. (Jr.), Mancall, E.L. Yakovlev, P.I.: The Human Cerebellum. An Atlas of Gross Topography in Serial Sections. Boston: Little and Brown 1961

9. Astruc, J.: Corticofugal connections of area 8 (frontal eye field) in Macaca mulatta. Brain Res. *33*, 241–256 (1971)

10. Baker, R., Berthoz, A.: Is the prepositus hypoglossi nucleus the source of another vestibulo-ocular pathway? Brain Res. *86*, 121–127 (1975)

11. Baker, R., Berthoz, A., Delgado-Garcia, J.: Monosynaptic excitation of trochlear motoneurons following electrical stimulation of the prepositus hypoglossi nucleus. Brain Res. *121*, 157–161 (1977)

12. Baker, R., Gresty, M., Berthoz, A.: Neuronal activity in the prepositus hypoglossi nucleus correlated with vertical and horizontal eye movement in the cat. Brain Res. *101*, 366–371 (1975)

13. Baker, R., Highstein, S.M.: Physiological identification of interneurons and motoneurons in the abducens nucleus. Brain Res. *91*, 292–298 (1975)

14. Baleydier, Chr.: A bilateral cortical projection to the superior colliculus in the cat. Neurosci. Lett. *4*, 9–14 (1977)

15. Batton, R.R., Jayaraman, A., Carpenter, M.B.: Fastigial projections in the monkey: an autoradiographic study. Anat. Rec. *187*, 532 (1977)

16. Beckstead, R.M.: Afferent connections of the entorhinal area as demonstrated by retrograde cell labeling with horseradish peroxidase. Anat. Rec. *187*, 534 (1977)

17. Benevento, L.A., Rezak, M., Santos-Anderson, R.: An autoradiographic study of the projections of the pretectum in the rhesus monkey (Macaca mulatta): Evidence for sensorimotor links to the thalamus an oculomotor nuclei. Brain Res. *127*, 197–218 (1977)

18. Benjamin, R.M., Burton, H.: Projection of taste nerve afferents to anterior opercular-insular cortex in squirrel monkey (Saimiri sciureus). Brain Res. *7*, 221–231 (1968)

19. Berrevoets, C.E., Kuypers, H.G.J.M.: Pericruciate cortical neurons projecting to brain stem reticular formation, dorsal column nuclei and spinal cord in the cat. Neurosci. Lett. *1*, 257–262 (1975)

20. Björklund, A., Lindvall, O., Nobin, A.: Evidence of an incertohypothalamic dopamine neurone system in the rat. Brain Res. *89*, 29–42 (1975)

21. Björklund, A., Nobin, A.: Fluorescence

histochemical and microspectrofluoromet-
ric mapping of dopamine and noradrenaline cell groups in the rat diencephalon.
Brain Res. *51*, 193–205 (1973)

22. Blackstad, T.W., Brink, K., Hem, J.,
Jeune, B.: Distribution of hippocampal
mossy fibers in rats. An experimental study
with silver impregnation methods. J.
Comp. Neurol. *138*, 433–450 (1970)

23. Bobillier, P., Seguin, S., Petitjean, F., Salvert, D., Touret, M., Jouvet, M.: The
raphe nuclei of the cat brain stem: a topographical atlas of their efferent projections as revealed by autoradiography.
Brain Res. *113*, 449–486 (1976)

24. Bowsher, D.: Some afferent and efferent
connections of the parafascicular-center
median complex. In: The Thalamus. Purpura, D.P., Yahr, M.D. (eds.). New York:
Columbia University Press 1966, pp.
99–108

25. Bowsher, D.: Introduction to the Anatomy and Physiology of the Nervous System. Oxford: Blackwell Scientific 1975a

26. Bowsher, D.: Diencephalic projections
from the midbrain reticular formation.
Brain Res. *95*, 211–220 (1975b)

27. Braak, H.: Über die Kerngebiete des
menschlichen Hirnstammes. II. Die
Raphekerne. Z. Zellforsch. *107*, 123–141
(1970)

28. Broadwell, R.D., Jacobowitz, D.M.: Olfactory relationships of the telencephalon
and diencephalon in the rabbit. III. The
ipsilateral centrifugal fibers to the olfactory bulbar and retrobulbar formations. J.
Comp. Neurol. *170*, 321–346 (1976)

29. Brodal, A.: Untersuchungen über die
Olivo-Cerebellaren Lokalisation. Z. Neurol. *169*, 1–53 (1940)

30. Brodal, A.: The reticular formation of the
brain stem. Anatomical aspects and functional correlations. Edinburgh: Oliver and
Boyd 1957

31. Brodal, A.: Neurological Anatomy in Relation to Clinical Medicine. New York-
London-Toronto: Oxford University Press
1969

32. Brown, J.T., Chan-Palay, V., Palay, S.L.:
A study of afferent input to the inferior
olivary complex in the rat by retrograde
axonal transport of horseradish peroxidase. J. Comp. Neurol. *176*, 1–22 (1977)

33. Brown, R.M., Goldman, P.S.: Catecholamines in neocortex of rhesus monkeys: re-
gional distribution and ontogenetic development. Brain Res. *124*, 576–580 (1977)

34. Carman, J.B., Cowan, W.M., Powell,
T.P.S.: The organization of the corticostriate connexions in the rabbit. Brain *86*,
525–562 (1963)

35. Carman, J.B., Cowan, W.M., Powell,
T.P.S.: Cortical connections of the thalamic reticular nucleus. J. Anat. (Lond.)
98, 587–598 (1964)

36. Carmel, P.W.: Efferent projections of the
ventral anterior nucleus of the thalamus
in the monkey. Am. J. Anat. *128*, 159–184
(1970)

37. Carpenter, M.B.: Human Neuroanatomy.
Baltimore: Williams and Wilkins 1976

38. Carpenter, M.B., Fraser, R.A.R., Shriver,
J.E.: The organization of pallidosubtha-
lamic fibers in the monkey. Brain Res. *11*,
522–559 (1968)

39. Carpenter, M.B., Harbison, J.W., Peter,
P.: Accessory oculomotor nuclei in the
monkey: projections and effects of discrete
lesions. J. Comp. Neurol. *140*, 131–154
(1970)

40. Carpenter, M.B., Nakano, K., Kim, R.:
Nigrothalamic projections in the monkey
demonstrated by autoradiographic tech-
nics. J. Comp. Neurol. *165*, 401–416 (1976)

41. Carpenter, M.B., Peter, Ph.: Nigrostriatal
and nigrothalamic fibers in the rhesus
monkey. J. Comp. Neurol. *144*, 93–117
(1972)

42. Catsman-Berrevoets, C.E., Kuypers,
H.G.J.M.: Cells of origin of cortical projections to dorsal column nuclei, spinal
cord and bulbar medial reticular formation
in the rhesus monkey. Neurosci. Lett. *3*,
245–252 (1976)

43. Chan-Palay, V.: Cerebellar Dentate Nucleus. Berlin-Heidelberg-New York:
Springer 1977

44. Chan-Palay, V.: Indoleamine neurons and
their processes in the normal rat brain and
in chronic diet-induced thiamine deficiency
demonstrated by uptake of ^{3}H-serotonin.
J. Comp. Neurol. *176*, 467–494 (1977)

45. Conrad, C.D., Stumpf, W.E.: Endocrine-
optic pathways to the hypothalamus. In:
Anatomical Neuroendocrinology. Int.
Conf. Neurobiology of CNS-Hormone In-

teractions, Chapel Hill 1974. Stumpf, W.E., Grant, L.D. (eds.). Basel: Karger 1975, pp. 15–29

46. Conrad, L.C.A., Leonard, Ch.M., Pfaff, D.W.: Connections of the median and dorsal raphe nuclei in the rat: an autoradiographic and degeneration study. J. Comp. Neurol. *156*, 179–206 (1974)

47. Conrad, L.C.A., Pfaff, D.W.: Efferents from medial basal forebrain and hypothalamus in the rat. I. An autoradiographic study of the medial preoptic area. J. Comp. Neurol. *169*, 185–220 (1976a)

48. Conrad, L.C.A., Pfaff, D.W.: Efferents from medial basal forebrain an hypothalamus in the rat. II. An autoradiographic study of the anterior hypothalamus. J. Comp. Neurol. *169*, 221–262 (1976b)

49. Cowan, W.M., Raisman, G., Powell, T.S.: The connexions of the amygdala. J. Neurol. Neurosurg. Psychiatry *28*, 137–151 (1965)

50. Crosby, E.C., Humphrey, T.: Studies of the vertebrate telencephalon. II. The nuclear pattern of the anterior olfactory nucleus, tuberculum olfactorium and the amygdaloid complex in adult man. J. Comp. Neurol. *47*, 309–352 (1941)

51. Crosby, E.C., Humphrey, T., Lauer, E.W.: Correlative Anatomy of the Nervous System. New York: MacMillan 1962

52. Crosby, E.C., Woodburne, R.T.: The comparative anatomy of the preoptic area and the hypothalamus. Res. Publ. Assoc. Res. Nerv. Ment. Dis. *20*, 52–169 (1940)

53. Cruce, J.A.F.: An autoradiographic study of the descending connections of the mammillary nuclei of the rat. J. Comp. Neurol. *176*, 631–644 (1977)

54. Crutcher, K.A.: An attempt to identify the suprasegmental source of spinal cord monoamines in the opossum (Didelphis marsupialis). Anat. Rec. *187*, 559 (1977)

55. Dahlström, A., Fuxe, K.: Evidence for the existence of monoamine-containing neurons in the central nervous system. I. Demonstration of monoamines in the cell bodies of brain stem neurons. Acta Physiol. Scand. *62* [suppl. 232], 1–55 (1964)

56. Dahlström, A., Fuxe, K.: Evidence for the existence of monoamine neurons in the central nervous system. II. Experimentally induced changes in the intraneuronal amine levels of bulbospinal neuron systems. Acta Physiol. Scand. *64* [Suppl. 247], 1–36 (1965)

57. Darian Smith, J.: The trigeminal system. In: Handbook of Sensory Physiology. Somatosensory system. Iggi, A. (ed.). Berlin-Heidelberg-New York: Springer 1973, pp. 271–314

58. Deecke, L., Schwarz, D.W.F., Fredrickson, J.M.: Nucleus ventroposterior inferior (VPI) as the vestibular thalamic relay in the rhesus monkey. I. Field potential investigation. Exp. Brain Res. *20*, 88–100 (1974)

59. Déjérine, J.: Anatomie des centres nerveux. Paris: Rueff 1895

60. Dennis, B.J., Kerr, D.I.B.: Origins of olfactory bulb centrifugal fibres in the cat. Brain Res. *110*, 593–600 (1976)

61. De Olmos, J.S.: The amygdaloid projection field in the rat as studied with the cupric-silver method. In: The Neurobiology of the Amygdala. Eleftheriou, B.E. (ed.). New York: Plenum Press 1972, pp. 145–204

62. Devito, J.L.: A horseradish peroxidase study of subcortical projections to the hippocampal formation in squirrel monkey (Saimiri sciureus). Neurosci. Abstr. *3*, p. 196 (1977)

63. Dewulf, A.: Anatomy of the Normal Human Thalamus. Amsterdam: Elsevier 1971

64. Domesick, V.B.: Projections from the cingulate cortex in the rat. Brain Res. *12*, 296–320 (1969)

65. Domesick, V.B.: The fasciculus cinguli in the rat. Brain Res. *20*, 19–32 (1970)

66. Domesick, V.B.: Projections of the nucleus of the diagonal band of Broca in the rat. Anat. Rec. *184*, 391–392 (1976)

67. Eccles, J.C., Ito, M., Szentágothai, J.: The Cerebellum as a Neuronal Machine. Berlin-Heidelberg-New York: Springer 1967

68. Edwards, S.B.: Autoradiographic studies of the projections of the midbrain reticular formation: descending projections of nucleus cuneiformis. J. Comp. Neurol. *161*, 341–358 (1975)

69. Edwards, S.B., De Olmos, J.S.: Autoradiographic studies of the projections of the midbrain reticular formation: ascending projections of nucleus cuneiformis. J. Comp. Neurol. *165*, 417–432 (1976)

70. Felten, D.L., Laties, A.M., Carpenter, M.B.: Monoamine-containing cell bodies in the squirrel monkey brain. Am. J. Anat. *139*, 153–166 (1974)

71. Fox, C.A., Rafols, J.A.: The radial fibers in the globus pallidus. J. Comp. Neurol. *159*, 177–200 (1975)

72. Fox, C.A., Rafols, J.A., Cowan, W.M.: Computer measurements of axis cylinder diameters of radial fibers and "comb" bundle fibers. J. Comp. Neurol. *159*, 201–224 (1975)

73. Fredrickson, J.M., Kornhuber, H.H., Schwarz, D.W.F.: Cortical projections of the vestibular nerve. In: Handbook of Sensory Physiology. Vol. VI,1: Vestibular System, part I: Basic Mechanisms. Kornhuber, H.H. (ed.). Berlin-Heidelberg-New York: Springer 1974, pp. 565–582

74. Fuxe, K., Jonsson, G.: Further mapping of central 5-hydroxytryptamine neurons: studies with the neurotoxic dihydroxytryptamines. In: Advances in Biochemical Psychopharmacology. Costa, E., Gessa, G.L., Sandler, M. (eds). New York: Raven Press 1974, Vol. 10, pp. 1–12

75. Garver, D.L., Sladek, J.R. (Jr.): Monoamine distribution in primate brain. I. Catecholamine-containing perikarya in the brain stem of Macaca speciosa. J. Comp. Neurol. *159*, 289–304 (1975)

76. Gaskell, W.H.: On the structure, distribution and function of the nerves which innervate the visceral and vascular systems. J. Physiol. *7*, 1–81 (1886)

77. Gaskell, W.H.: On the relation between the structure, function, distribution and origin of the cranial nerves; together with a theory of the origin of the nervous system of vertebrata. J. Physiol. *10*, 153–211 (1889)

78. Gatter, K.C., Powell, T.P.S.: The projection of the locus coeruleus upon the neocortex in the macaque monkey. Neuroscience *2*, 441–445 (1977)

79. Geyer, M.A., Puerto, A., Dawsey, W.J., Knapp, S., Bullard, W.P., Mandell, A.J.: Histologic and enzymatic studies of the mesolimbic and mesostriatal serotonergic pathways. Brain Res. *106*, 241–256 (1976)

80. Graybiel, A.M.: Direct and indirect preoculomotor pathways of the brainstem: an autoradiographic study of the pontine reticular formation in the cat. J. Comp. Neurol. *175*, 37–78 (1977)

81. Graybiel, A.M., Hartwieg, E.A.: Some afferent connections of the oculomotor complex in the cat: an experimental study with tracer techniques. Brain Res. *81*, 543–551 (1974)

82. Graybiel, A.M., Sciascia, T.R.: Origin and distribution of nigrotectal fibers in the cat. Neurosci. Abs. *1*, 174 (1975)

83. Groenewegen, H.J., Voogd, J.: The parasagittal zonation within the olivocerebellar projection. I. Climbing fiber distribution in the vermis of cat cerebellum. J. Comp. Neurol. *174*, 417–488 (1977)

84. Grofová, I., Rinvik, E.: An experimental electron microscopic study on the striatonigral projection in the cat. Exp. Brain Res. *11*, 249–262 (1970)

85. Halász, N., Ljungdahl, A., Hökfelt, T., Johansson, O., Goldstein, M., Park, D., Biberfeld, P.: Transmitter histochemistry of the rat olfactory bulb. I. Immunohistochemical localization of monoamine synthesizing enzymes. Support for intrabulbar periglomerular dopamine neurons. Brain Res. *126*, 455–474 (1977)

86. Hancock, M.B.: Cells of origin of hypothalamo-spinal projections in the rat. Neurosci. Lett. *3*, 179–184 (1976)

87. Harting, J.K., Hall, W.C., Diamond, I.T.: Projections from the visual thalamus to neocortex in the tree shrew (Tupaia glis). Anat. Rec. *169*, 335 (1971).

88. Hartman, B.K.: The innervation of cerebral blood vessels by central noradrenergic neurons. In: Frontiers in Catecholamine Research. Usdin, E., Snyder, S.H., (eds.). Oxford: Pergamon Press 1973, pp. 91–96

89. Hartman, B.K., Zide, D., Udenfriend, S.: The use of dopamine β-hydroxylase as a marker for the central noradrenergic nervous system in rat brain. Proc. Nat. Acad. Sci. USA *69*, 2722–2726 (1972)

90. Hassler, R.: Anatomy of the thalamus. In: Introduction to Stereotaxis with an Atlas of the Human Brain. Schaltenbrand, G., Bailey, P., (eds.). Stuttgart: Thieme 1959, pp. 230–290

91. Heimer, L.: The olfactory connections of the diencephalon in the rat. An experimental light and electron microscopic study with special emphasis on the problem of terminal degeneration. Brain Behav. Evol. *6*, 484–523 (1972)

92. Heimer, L.: Olfactory projections to the diencephalon. In: Anatomical Neuroendocrinology. Int. Conf. Neurobiology of CNS-Hormone Interactions, Chapel Hill 1974. Stumpf, W.E., Grant, L.D., (eds.). Basel: Karger 1975, pp. 30–39

93. Heimer, L., Nauta, W.J.H.: The hypothalamic distribution of the stria terminalis in the rat. Brain Res. *13*, 284–297 (1969)

94. Herkenham, M., Nauta, W.J.H.: Afferent connections of the habenular nuclei in the rat. A horseradish peroxidase study, with a note on the fiber-of-passage problem. J. Comp. Neurol. *173*, 123–146 (1977a)

95. Herkenham, M., Nauta, W.J.H.: Projections of the habenular nuclei in the rat. Anat. Rec. *187*, 603 (1977b)

96. Herrick, C.J.: Anatomy of the brain. In: The Reference Handbook of the Medical Sciences. New York: Wood 1913, Vol. 2, pp. 274–342

97. Herzog, A.G., Van Hoesen, G.W.: Temporal neocortical afferent connections to the amygdala in the rhesus monkey. Brain Res. *115*, 57–69 (1976)

98. Highstein, S.M., Maekawa, K., Steinacker, A., Cohen, B.: Synaptic input from the pontine reticular nuclei to abducens motoneurons and internuclear neurons in the cat. Brain Res. *112*, 162–167 (1976)

99. Hjorth-Simonsen, A.: Hippocampal efferents to the ipsilateral entorhinal area: an experimental study in the rat. J. Comp. Neurol. *142*, 417–438 (1971)

100. Hjorth-Simonsen, A.: Projection of the lateral part of the entorhinal area to the hippocampus area and fascia dentata. J. Comp. Neurol. *146*, 219–232 (1972)

101. Hjorth-Simonsen, A.: Some intrinsic connections of the hippocampus in the rat: An experimental analysis. J. Comp. Neurol. *147*, 163–180 (1973)

102. Hoddevik, G.H., Brodal, A., Walberg, F.: The reticulovestibular projection in the cat. An experimental study with silver impregnation methods. Brain Res. *94*, 383–399 (1975)

103. Holländer, H.: On the origin of the corticotectal projections in the cat. Exp. Brain Res. *21*, 433–439 (1974)

104. Holstege, G., Kuypers, H.G.J.M.: Propriobulbar fibre connections to the trigeminal, facial and hypoglossal motor nuclei. I. An anterograde degeneration study in the cat. Brain *100*, 239–264 (1977)

105. Holstege, G., Kuypers, H.G.J.M., Dekker, J.J.: The organization of the bulbar fibre connections to the trigeminal, facial and hypoglossal motor nuclei. II. An autoradiographic tracing study in cat. Brain *100*, 265–286 (1977)

105a. Hopkins, D.A.: Amygdalotegmental projections in the rat, cat and rhesus monkey. Neurosci. Letters, *1*, 263–270 (1975)

106. Hopkins, D.A., Niessen, L.W.: Substantia nigra projections to the reticular formation, superior colliculus and central gray in the rat, cat and monkey. Neurosci. Lett. *2*, 253–259 (1976)

107. Hubbard, J.E., Di Carlo, V.: Fluorescence histochemistry of monoamine-containing cell bodies in the brain stem of the squirrel monkey (Saimiri sciureus). I. The locus caeruleus. J. Comp. Neurol. *147*, 553–566 (1973)

108. Hubbard, J.E., Di Carlo, V.: Fluorescence histochemistry of monoamine-containing cell bodies in the brain stem of the squirrel monkey (Saimiri sciureus). II. Catecholamine-containing groups. J. Comp. Neurol. *153*, 369–384 (1974)

109. Hubbard, J.E., Di Carlo, V.: Fluorescence histochemistry of monoamine-containing cell bodies in the brain stem of the squirrel monkey (Saimiri sciureus). III. Serotonin-containing groups. J. Comp. Neurol. *153*, 385–398 (1974)

110. Ito, M.: Cerebellar learning control of vestibulo-ocular mechanisms. In: Mechanisms in Transmission of Signals for Conscious Behavior. Desiraju, T. (ed.). Amsterdam: Elsevier 1976, pp. 1–22

111. Jacobowitz, D.M.: Fluorescence microscopic mapping of CNS norepinephrine systems in the rat forebrain. In: Anatomical Neuroendocrinology. Stumpf, W.E., Grant, L.D. (eds.). Basel: Karger 1975, pp. 368–380

112. Jacobson, S., Trojanowski, J.Q.: The cells of origin of the corpus callosum in rat, cat and rhesus monkey. Brain Res. *74*, 149–155 (1974)

113. Jacobson, S., Trojanowski, J.Q.: Amygdaloid projections to prefrontal granular cortex in rhesus monkey demonstrated with horseradish peroxidase. Brain Res. *100*, 132–139 (1975)

114. Jelgersma, G.: Atlas Anatomicum Cerebri Humani. Amsterdam: Scheltema and Holkema N.V. 1931

115. Jones, B.E., Moore, R.Y.: Ascending projections of the locus coeruleus in the rat. II. Autoradiographic study. Brain Res. *127*, 23–53 (1977)

116. Jones, E.G.: Some aspects of the organization of the thalamic reticular complex. J. Comp. Neurol. *162*, 285–308 (1975)

117. Jones, E.G., Leavitt, R.Y.: Retrograde axonal transport and the demonstration of non-specific projections to the cerebral cortex an striatum from thalamic intralaminar nuclei in the cat, rat and monkey. J. Comp. Neurol. *154*, 349–378 (1974)

118. Jones, E.G., Powell, T.P.S.: Connexions of the somatic sensory cortex of the rhesus monkey. I. Ipsilateral cortical connexions. Brain *92*, 447–502 (1969)

119. Jones, E.G., Wise, S.P.: Size, laminar and columnar distribution of efferent cells in the sensory-motor cortex of monkeys. J. Comp. Neurol. *175*, 391–438 (1977)

120. Kasdon, D.L., Jacobson, S.: The thalamic afferents to the inferior parietal lobule of the rhesus monkey. J. Comp. Neurol. *177*, 685–706 (1978)

121. Kemp, J.M., Powell, T.P.S.: The corticostriate projection in the monkey. Brain *93*, 525–547 (1970)

122. Kemper, T.L.: The organization and connections of the human septum and septal area. Anat. Rec. *184*, 444 (1976)

123. Kerr, F.W.L.: Neuroanatomical substrates of nociception in the spinal cord. Pain *1*, 325–356 (1975)

124. Kerr, F.W.L., Lippmann, H.H.: The primate spinothalamic tract as demonstrated by anterolateral cordotomy and commissural myelotomy. In: International Symposium on Pain. Advances in Neurology. Bonica, J.J. (ed.). New York: Raven Press 1974, Vol. 4, pp. 147–156

125. Kievit, J., Kuypers, H.G.J.M.: Organization of the thalamo-cortical connexions to the frontal lobe in the rhesus monkey. Exp. Brain Res. *29*, 299–322 (1977)

126. Kim, R., Nakano, K., Jayaraman, A., Carpenter, B.: Projections of the globus pallidus and adjacent structures: an autoradiographic study in the monkey. J. Comp. Neurol. *169*, 263–290 (1976)

127. Koikegami, H.: Amygdala and other related limbic structures; experimental studies on the anatomy and function. I. Anatomical researches with some neurophysiological observations. Acta Med. Biol. *10*, 161–277 (1963)

128. Kotchabhakdi, N., Hoddevik, G.H., Walberg, F.: Cerebellar afferent projections from the perihypoglossal nuclei: an experimental study with the method of retrograde axonal transport of horseradish peroxidase. Exp. Brain Res. *31*, 13–29 (1978)

129. Köves, K., Réthelyi, M.: Direct neural connection from the medial preoptic area to the hypothalamic arcuate nucleus of the rat. Exp. Brain Res. *25*, 529–539 (1976)

130. Krettek, J.E., Price, J.L.: A direct input from the amygdala to the thalamus and the cerebral cortex. Brain Res. *67*, 169–174 (1974a)

131. Krettek, J.E., Price, J.L.: Projections from the amygdala to the perirhinal and entorhinal cortices and the subiculum. Brain Res. *71*, 150–154 (1974b)

132. Krettek, J.E., Price, J.L.: Projections from the amygdaloid complex to the cerebral cortex and thalamus in the rat and cat. J. Comp. Neurol. *172*, 687–722 (1977a)

133. Krettek, J.E., Price, J.L.: Projections from the amygdaloid complex and adjacent olfactory structures to the entorhinal cortex and to the subiculum in the rat and cat. J. Comp. Neurol. *172*, 723–752 (1977b)

134. Krieger, M.S., Conrad, L.C.A., Pfaff, D.W.: Axonal projections from the ventromedial nucleus of the hypothalamus. Anat. Rec. *187*, 770–771 (1977)

135. Künzle, H., Akert, K.: Efferent connections of cortical, area 8 (frontal eye field) in Macaca fascicularis. A reinvestigation using the autoradiographic technique. J. Comp. Neurol. *173*, 147–164 (1977)

136. Kuo, J.S., Carpenter, M.B.: Organization of pallidothalamic projections in the rhesus monkey. J. Comp. Neurol. *151*, 201–236 (1973)

137. Kuypers, H.G.J.M.: Corticobulbar connections to the pons and lower brain-stem in man. Brain *81*, 364–388 (1958a)

138. Kuypers, H.G.J.M.: Some projections from the peri-central cortex to the pons and lower brain stem in monkey and chim-

panzee. J. Comp. Neurol. *110*, 221–256 (1958b)

139. Kuypers, H.G.J.M.: Central cortical projections to motor and somatosensory cell groups. Brain *83*, 161–184 (1960)

140. Kuypers, H.G.J.M.: Discussion. In: The Thalamus. Purpura, D.P., Yahr, M.D. (eds.). New York: Columbia University Press 1966, pp. 122–126

141. Kuypers, H.G.J.M.: The anatomical organization of the descending pathways and their contributions to motor control especially in primates. In: New Developments in EMG and Clinical Neurophysiology. Desmedt, J.E. (ed.). Basel: Karger 1973, Vol. 3, pp. 38–68

142. Kuypers, H.G.J.M., Fleming, W.R., Farinholt, J.W.: Subcortical spinal projections in the rhesus monkey. J. Comp. Neurol. *118*, 107–137 (1962)

143. Kuypers, H.G.J.M., Lawrence, D.G.: Cortical projections to the red nucleus and the brain stem in the rhesus monkey. Brain Res. *4*, 151–188 (1967)

144. Kuypers, H.G.J.M., Szwarcbart, M.K., Mishkin, M., Rosvold, H.E.: Occipitotemporal corticocortical connections in the rhesus monkey. Exp. Neurol. *11*, 245–262 (1965)

145. Lammers, H.J.: The neural connections of the amygdaloid complex in mammals. In: The Neurobiology of the Amygdala. Eleftheriou, B.E. (ed.). New York: Plenum 1972, pp. 123–144

146. LaMotte, C.: Distribution of the tract of Lissauer and the dorsal root fibers in the primate spinal cord. J. Comp. Neurol. *172*, 529–561 (1977)

147. Larsell, O., Jansen, J.: The comparative anatomy and histology of the cerebellum. III. The human cerebellum, cerebellar connections, and cerebellar cortex. Minneapolis: University of Minnesota Press 1972

148. Lawrence, D.G., Kuypers, H.G.J.M.: The functional organization of the motor system in the monkey. I. The effects of bilateral pyramidal lesions. Brain *91*, 1–14 (1968a)

149. Lawrence, D.G., Kuypers, H.G.J.M.: The functional organization of the motor system in the monkey. II. The effects of lesions of the descending brain-stem pathways. Brain *91*, 15–36 (1968b)

150. Leichnetz, G.R., Astruc, J.: The course of some prefrontal corticofugals to the pallidum, substantia innominata, and amygdaloid complex in monkeys. Exp. Neurol. *54*, 104–109 (1977)

151. Leonard, C.M., Scott, J.W.: Origin and distribution of the amygdalofugal pathways in the rat: an experimental neuroanatomical study. J. Comp. Neurol. *141*, 313–330 (1971)

152. Lindvall, O.: Mesencephalic dopamine afferents to the lateral septal nucleus of the rat. Brain Res. *87*, 89–95 (1975)

153. Lindvall, O., Björklund, A., Moore, R.Y., Stenevi, U.: Mesencephalic dopamine neurons projecting to neocortex. Brain Res. *81*, 325–331 (1974)

154. Lindvall, O., Björklund, A., Nobin, A., Stenevi, U.: The adrenergic innervation of the rat thalamus as revealed by the glyoxylic acid fluorescence method. J. Comp. Neurol. *154*, 317–348 (1974)

155. Llamas, A., Avendano, C., Reinoso-Suarez, F.: Amygdaloid projections to prefrontal and motor cortex. Science *195*, 794–796 (1977)

156. Lund, J.S., Lund, R.D., Hendrickson, A.E., Bunt, A.H., Fuchs, A.F.: The origin of efferent pathways from the primary visual cortex, area 17, of the macaque monkey as shown by retrograde transport of horseradish peroxidase. J. Comp. Neurol. *164*, 287–304 (1975)

157. Maciewicz, R.J., Eagen, K., Kaneko, C.R.S., Highstein, S.M.: Vestibular and medullary brain stem afferents to the abducens nucleus in the cat. Brain Res. *123*, 229–240 (1977)

158. Maciewicz, R.J., Kaneko, C.R.S., Highstein, S.M., Baker, R.: Morphophysiological identification of interneurons in the oculomotor nucleus that project to the abducens nucleus in the cat. Brain Res. *96*, 60–65 (1975)

159. McBride, R.L., Sutin, J.: Amygdaloid and pontine projections to the ventromedial nucleus of the hypothalamus. J. Comp. Neurol. *174*, 377–396 (1977)

160. Mehler, W.R.: The anatomy of the so-called "pain tract" in man: An analysis of the course and distribution of the ascending fibers of the fasciculus anterolateralis. In: Basic Research in Paraplegia.

French, J.D., Porter, R.W. (eds.). Springfield (Illinois): Thomas 1962, pp. 26–55

161. Mehler, W.R.: Further notes on the centre médian, nucleus of Luys. In: The Thalamus. Purpura, D.P., Yahr, M.D. (eds.). New York: Columbia University Press 1966a, pp. 109–127

162. Mehler, W.R.: The posterior thalamic region in man. Confin. Neurol. *27*, 18–29 (1966b)

163. Mehler, W.R.: Some neurological species differences – a posteriori. Ann. N.Y. Acad. Sci. *167*, 424–468 (1969)

164. Mehler, W.R.: Idea of a new anatomy of the thalamus. J. Psychiatr. Res. *8*, 203–217 (1971)

165. Mehler, W.R., Nauta, W.J.H.: Connections of the basal ganglia and of the cerebellum. Confin. Neurol. *36*, 205–222 (1974)

166. Meibach, R.C., Siegel, A.: The origin of fornix fibers which project to the mammillary bodies in the rat: a horseradish peroxidase study. Brain Res. *88*, 508–512 (1975)

167. Meibach, R.C., Siegel, A.: Efferent connections of the septal area in the rat: an analysis utilizing retrograde and anterograde transport methods. Brain Res. *119*, 1–20 (1977)

168. Molenaar, I., Kuypers, H.G.J.M.: Identification of cells of origin of long fiber connections in the cat's spinal cord by means of the retrograde axonal peroxidase technique. Neurosci. Lett. *1*, 193–197 (1975)

169. Montero, V.M., Guillery, R.W., Woolsey, C.N.: Retinotopic organization within the thalamic reticular nucleus demonstrated by a double label autoradiographic technique. Brain Res. *138*, 407–421 (1977)

170. Moore, R.Y.: Retinohypothalamic projection in mammals: a comparative study. Brain Res. *49*, 403–409 (1973)

171. Moore, R.Y.: Catecholamine innervation of the basal forebrain. I. The septal area. J. Comp. Neurol. *177*, 665–684 (1978)

172. Moore, R.Y., Halaris, A.E.: Hippocampal innervation by serotonin neurons of the midbrain raphe in the rat. J. Comp. Neurol. *164*, 171–183 (1975)

173. Morest, D.K.: Connexions of the dorsal tegmental nucleus in rat and rabbit. J. Anat (Lond.) *95*, 229–246 (1961)

174. Morest, D.K.: Experimental study of the projections of the nucleus of the tractus solitarius and the area postrema in the cat. J. Comp. Neurol. *130*, 277–300 (1967)

175. Motokizawa, F., Furuya, N.: Neural pathway associated with the EEG arousal response by olfactory stimulation. Electroencephalogr. Clin. Neurophysiol. *35*, 83–92 (1973)

176. Nauta, H.J.W.: Evidence of a pallidohabenular pathway in the cat. J. Comp. Neurol. *156*, 19–27 (1974)

177. Nauta. H.J.W., Cole, M.: Efferent projections of the subthalamic nucleus. Trans. Am. Neurol. Assoc. *99*, 170–173 (1974)

178. Nauta, W.J.H.: An experimental study of the fornix in the rat. J. Comp. Neurol. *104*, 247–272 (1956)

179. Nauta, W.J.H.: Hippocampal projections and related neural pathways to the midbrain in the cat. Brain *81*, 319–340 (1958)

180. Nauta, W.J.H.: Fibre degeneration following lesions of the amygdaloid complex in the monkey. J. Anat. (Lond.) *95*, 515–531 (1961)

181. Nauta, W.J.H.: Neural associations of the amygdaloid complex in the monkey. Brain *85*, 505–519 (1962)

182. Nauta, W.J.H.: The central visceromotor system: a general survey. In: Limbic System Mechanics and Autonomic Function. Hockman, Ch.C. (ed.). Springfield (Illinois): Thomas 1972, pp. 21–38

183. Nauta, W.J.H., Haymaker, W.: Hypothalamic nuclei and fiber connections. In: The Hypothalamus. Haymaker, W., Anderson, E., Nauta, W.J.H. (eds). Springfield (Illinois): Thomas 1969, pp. 136–209

184. Nauta, W.J.H., Kuypers, H.G.J.M.: Some ascending pathways in the brain stem reticular formation. In: Reticular Formation of the Brain. Jasper, H.H. and Proctor, L.D. (eds.). Toronto: Little and Brown 1958, pp. 3–31

185. Nauta, W.J.H., Mehler, W.R.: Projections of the lentiform nucleus in the monkey. Brain Res. *1*, 3–42 (1966)

186. Nieuwenhuys, R.: Topological analysis of the brain stem: a general introduction. J. Comp. Neurol. *156*, 255–276 (1974)

187. Nieuwenhuys, R.: Aspects of the morphology of the striatum. In: Psychobiology of the Striatum. Cools, A.R., Lohman, A.H.M., van den Bercken, J.H.L. (eds.). Amsterdam: Elsevier 1977, pp. 1–19

188. Nobin, A., Björklund, A: Topography of the monoamine neuron systems in the human brain as revealed in fetuses. Acta Physiol. Scand. [suppl.] *388*, 1–40 (1973)

189. Nomina Anatomica. Amsterdam: Excerpta Medica Foundation 1968.

190. Norgren, R.E.: Taste pathways to hypothalamus and amygdala. J. Comp. Neurol. *166*, 17–30 (1976)

191. Norgren, R.E., Leonard, C.M.: Taste pathways in rat brain stem. Science *173*, 1136–1139 (1971)

192. Norgren, R.E., Leonard, C.M.: Ascending central gustatory pathways. J. Comp. Neurol. *150*, 217–238 (1973)

193. Nygren, L.-G., Olson, L.: A new major projection from locus coeruleus: the main source of noradrenergic nerve terminals in the ventral and dorsal columns of the spinal cord. Brain Res. *132*, 85–93 (1977)

194. Olson, L., Fuxe, K.: On the projections from the locus coeruleus noradrenaline neurons: The cerebellar innervation. Brain Res. *28*, 165–171 (1971)

195. Olszewski, J.: The Thalamus of the Macaca Mulatta. Basel: Karger 1952.

196. Olszewski, J., Baxter, D.: Cytoarchitecture of the Human Brain Stem. Basel: Karger 1954

197. Palay, S.L., Chan-Palay, V.: Cerebellar Cortex. Cytology and Organization. Berlin-Heidelberg-New York: Springer 1974

198. Palkovits, M., Saavedra, J.M., Jacobowitz, D.M., Kizer, J.S., Zaborszky, L., Brownstein, M.J.: Serotonergic innervation of the forebrain: effect of lesions on serotonin and tryptophan hydroxylase levels. Brain Res. *130*, 121–134 (1977)

199. Pandya, D.N., Hallet, M., Mukherjee, S.K.: Intra- and interhemispheric connections of the neocortical auditory system in the rhesus monkey. Brain Res. *14*, 49–65 (1969)

200. Pandya, D.N., Karol, E.A., Heilbronn, D.: The topographical distribution of interhemispheric projections in the corpus callosum of the rhesus monkey. Brain Res. *32*, 31–43 (1971)

201. Pandya, D.N., Karol, E.A., Padmakar, P.L.: The distribution of the anterior commissure in the squirrel monkey. Brain Res. *49*, 177–180 (1973)

202. Pandya, D.N., Kuypers, H.G.J.M.: Cortico-cortical connections in the rhesus monkey. Brain Res. *13*, 13–36 (1969)

203. Pandya, D.N., Van Hoesen, G.W., Domesick, V.B.: A cingulo-amygdaloid projection in the rhesus monkey. Brain Res. *61*, 369–373 (1973)

204. Pandya, D.N., Vignolo, L.A.: Interhemispheric projections of the parietal lobe in the rhesus monkey. Brain Res. *15*, 49–65 (1969)

205. Papez, J.W.: A proposed mechanism of emotion. Arch. Neurol. Psychiatry *38*, 725–743 (1937)

206. Pasquier, D.A.: Evidence of direct projections from the centralis superior, dorsalis raphe and locus coeruleus nuclei to dorsal and ventral hippocampus in the cat. Anat. Rec. *184*, 498 (1976)

207. Pasquier, D.A., Forbes, W.B., Kemper, T.L., Morgane, P.J.: Serotonergic (dorsalis raphe nucleus) connections with the striatum. Anat. Rec. *187*, 677 (1977)

208. Pasquier, D.A., Reinoso-Suarez, F.: Differential efferent connections of the brain stem to the hippocampus in the cat. Brain Res. *120*, 540–548 (1977)

209. Petras, J.M.: Some efferent connections of the motor and somatosensory cortex of simian primates and felid, canid and procyonid carnivores. Ann. N.Y. Acad. Sci. *167*, 469–505 (1969)

210. Powell, T.P.S., Cowan, W.M., Raisman, G.: The central olfactory connexions. J. Anat. (Lond.) *99*, 791–813 (1965)

211. Raichle, M.E., Hartman, B.K., Eichling, J.O., Sharpe, L.G.: Central noradrenergic regulation of cerebral blood flow and vascular permeability. Proc. Nat. Acad. Sci. USA *72*, 3726–3730 (1975)

212. Raymond, J., Sans, A., Marty, R.: Projections thalamiques des noyaux vestibulaires: étude histologique chez le chat. Exp. Brain Res. *20*, 273–283 (1974)

213. Renaud, L.P., Hopkins, D.A.: Amygdala afferents from the mediobasal hypothalamus: an electrophysiological and neuroanatomical study in the rat. Brain Res. *121*, 201–213 (1977)

214. Rhoton, A.L.: Afferent connections of the facial nerve. J. Comp. Neurol. *133*, 89–100 (1968)

215. Ricardo, J.A., Koh, E.T.: Direct projections from the nucleus of the solitary tract

to the hypothalamus, amygdala, and other forebrain structures in the rat. Anat. Rec. *187*, 693 (1977)

216. Riley, H.A.: An Atlas of the Basal Ganglia, Brain Stem and Spinal Cord. New York: Hafner 1960

217. Rinvik, E.: Demonstration of nigrothalamic connections in the cat by retrograde axonal transport of horseradish peroxidase. Brain Res. *90*, 313–318 (1975)

218. Rinvik, E., Grofová, I., Ottersen, O.P.: Demonstration of nigrotectal and nigroreticular projections in the cat by axonal transport of proteins. Brain Res. *112*, 388–394 (1976)

219. Rosene, D.L., Heimer, L.: Olfactory bulb efferents in the rhesus monkey. Anat. Rec. *187*, 698 (1977)

220. Rosene, D.L., Van Hoesen, G.W.: Hippocampal efferents reach widespread areas of cerebral cortex and amygdala in the rhesus monkey. Science *198*, 315–317 (1977)

221. Sakai, K., Touret, M., Salvert, D., Leger, L., Jouvet, M.: Afferent projections to the cat locus coeruleus as visualized by the horseradish peroxidase technique. Brain Res. *119*, 21–41 (1977)

222. Saper, C.B., Loewy, A.D., Swanson, L.W., Cowan, W.M.: Direct hypothalamo-autonomic connections. Brain Res. *117*, 305–312 (1976)

223. Saper, C.B., Swanson, L.W., Cowan, W.M.: The efferent connections of the ventromedial nucleus of the hypothalamus of the rat. J. Comp. Neurol. *169*, 409–442 (1976)

224. Satoh, K., Tohyama, M., Yamamoto, K., Sakumoto, T., Shimizu, N.: Noradrenaline innervation of the spinal cord studied by the horseradish peroxidase method combined with monoamine oxidase staining. Exp. Brain Res. *30*, 175–186 (1977)

225. Schaltenbrand, G., Bailey, P.: Einführung in die stereotaktischen Operationen mit einem Atlas des menschlichen Gehirns. 3 Vols. Stuttgart: Thieme 1959

226. Schoen, J.R.: Comparative aspects of the descending fibre systems in the spinal cord. In: Progress in Brain Research. Eccles, J.C., Schadé, J.P. (eds.). Amsterdam: Elsevier 1964, Vol. 11, pp. 203–222

227. Scott, J.W., Leonard, C.M.: The olfactory connections of the lateral hypothalamus in the rat, mouse and hamster. J. Comp. Neurol. *141*, 331–345 (1971)

228. Shipley, M.T.: Presubiculum afferents to the entorhinal area and the Papez circuit. Brain Res. *67*, 162–168 (1974)

229. Shipley, M.T.: The topographical and laminar organization of the presubiculum's projection to the ipsi- and contralateral entorhinal cortex in the guinea pig. J. Comp. Neurol. *160*, 127–145 (1975)

230. Shipley, M.T., Sörensen, K.E.: On the laminar organization of the anterior thalamus projections to the presubiculum in the guinea pig. Brain Res. *86*, 473–477 (1975)

231. Sie, P.G.: Localization of Fibre Systems Within the White Matter of the Medulla Oblongata and the Cervical Cord in Man. Thesis, Leiden (1956)

232. Singer, M., Yakovlev, P.I.: The human brain in sagittal section. Springfield (Illinois): Thomas 1954

233. Smith, R.L.: Axonal projections and connections of the principal sensory trigeminal nucleus in the monkey. J. Comp. Neurol. *163*, 347–376 (1975)

234. Spatz, W.B.: An efferent connection of the solitary cells of Meynert. A study with horseradish peroxidase in the marmoset Callithrix. Brain Res. *92*, 450–455 (1975)

235. Stephan, H.: Handbuch der mikroskopischen Anatomie des Menschen. Vol. 4, Part 9: Allocortex. Berlin-Heidelberg-New York: Springer 1975

236. Strominger, N.L., Nelson, L.R., Dougherty, W.J.: Second order auditory pathways in the chimpanzee. J. Comp. Neurol. *172*, 349–366 (1977)

237. Swanson, L.W.: The locus coeruleus: a cytoarchitectonic, Golgi and immunohistochemical study in the albino rat. Brain Res. *110*, 39–56 (1976)

238. Swanson, L.W.: An autoradiographic study of the efferent connections of the preoptic region in the rat. J. Comp. Neurol. *167*, 227–256 (1976)

239. Swanson, L.W., Connelly, M.A., Hartman, B.K.: Ultrastructural evidence for central monoaminergic innervation of blood vessels in the paraventricular nucleus of the hypothalamus. Brain Res. *136*, 166–173 (1977)

240. Swanson, L.W., Cowan, W.M.: Hippo-

campo-hypothalamic connections: origin in subicular cortex, not Ammon's horn. Science *189*, 303–304 (1975)

241. Swanson, L.W., Cowan, W.M.: An autoradiographic study of the organization of the efferent connections of the hippocampal formation in the rat. J. Comp. Neurol. *172*, 49–84 (1977)

242. Swanson, L.W., Hartman, B.K.: The central adrenergic system, an immunofluorescence study of the location of cell bodies and their efferent connections in the rat utilizing dopamine-β-hydroxylase as a marker. J. Comp. Neurol. *163*, 467–506 (1975)

243. Szabo, J.: Projections from the body of the caudate nucleus in the rhesus monkey. Exp. Neurol. *27*, 1–15 (1970)

244. Taber, E., Brodal, A., Walberg, F.: The raphe nuclei of the brain stem in the cat. I. Normal topography and cytoarchitecture and general discussion. J. Comp. Neurol. *114*, 161–187 (1960)

245. Taber Pierce, E., Foote, W.E., Hobson, J.A.: The efferent connection of the nucleus raphe dorsalis. Brain Res. *107*, 137–144 (1976)

246. Tigges, J., Bos, J., Tigges, M.: An autoradiographic investigation of the subcortical visual system in chimpanzee. J. Comp. Neurol. *172*, 367–380 (1977)

247. Tohyama, M., Maeda, T., Shimizu, N.: Detailed noradrenaline pathways of locus coeruleus neuron to the cerebral cortex with use of 6-hydroxydopa. Brain Res. *79*, 139–144 (1974)

248. Tolbert, D.L., Bantli, H., Bloedel, J.R.: Anatomical and physiological evidence for a cerebellar nucleo-cortical projection in the cat. Neuroscience *1*, 205–217 (1976)

249. Torvik, A.: The ascending fibers from the main trigeminal sensory nucleus. An experimental study in the cat. Am. J. Anat. *100*, 1–16 (1957a)

250. Torvik, A.: The spinal projection from the nucleus of the solitary tract. An experimental study in the cat. J. Anat. (Lond.) *91*, 314–322 (1957b)

251. Trevino, D.L., Carstens, E.: Confirmation of the location of spinothalamic neurons in the cat and monkey by the retrograde transport of horseradish peroxidase. Brain Res. *98*, 177–182 (1975)

252. Troiano, R., Siegel, A: The ascending and descending connections of the hypothalamus in the cat. Exp. Neurol. *49*, 161–173 (1975)

253. Turner, B.H., Gupta, K.C., Mishkin, M.: The locus and cytoarchitecture of the projection areas of the olfactory bulb in Macaca mulatta. J. Comp. Neurol. *177*, 381–396 (1978)

254. Ungerstedt, U.: Stereotaxic mapping of the monoamine pathways in the rat brain. Acta Physiol. Scand. [suppl.] *367*, 1–49 (1971)

255. Updyke, B.V.: Topographic organization of the projections from cortical areas 17, 18 and 19 onto the thalamus, pretectum and superior colliculus in the cat. J. Comp. Neurol. *173*, 81–122 (1977)

256. Valverde, F.: Studies on the Piriform Lobe. Cambridge: Harvard University Press 1965

257. Van Buren, J.M., Borke, R.C.: Variations and Connections of the Human Thalamus. 2 Vols. Berlin-Heidelberg-New York: Springer 1972.

258. Van Hoesen, G.W., Pandya, D.N.: Some connections of the entorhinal area (area 28) and perirhinal area (area 35) cortices of the rhesus monkey. I. Temporal lobe afferents. Brain Res. *95*, 1–24 (1975)

259. Van Hoesen, G.W., Pandya, D.N., Butters, M.: Cortical afferents of the entorhinal cortex of the rhesus monkey. Science *175*, 1471–1473 (1972)

260. Van Hoesen, G.W., Pandya, D.N., Butters, M.: Some connections of the entorhinal area (area 28) and perirhinal area (area 35) cortices of the thesus monkey. II. Frontal afferents. Brain Res. *95*, 25–38 (1975)

261. Vogt, B.A., Pandya, D.N.: Cortico-cortical connections of somatic sensory cortex (areas 3, 1 and 2) in the rhesus monkey. J. Comp. Neurol. *177*, 179–192 (1977)

262. Voogd, J.: The Cerebellum of the Cat. Assen: Van Gorcum 1964

263. Voogd, J.: Comparative aspects of the structure and fibre connexions of the mammalian cerebellum. In: Progress in Brain Research. Fox, C.A., Snider, R.S. (eds.). Amsterdam: Elsevier 1967, Vol. 25, pp. 94–135

264. Walberg, F.: Fastigiofugal fibers to the

perihypoglossal nuclei in the cat. Exp. Neurol. *3*, 525–541 (1961)

265. Walker, A.E.: The Primate Thalamus. Chicago: University Press 1938

266. Wang, R.Y., Aghajanian, G.K.: Inhibition of neurons in the amygdala by dorsal raphe stimulation: mediation through a direct serotonergic pathway. Brain Res. *120*, 85–102 (1977)

267. Whitlock, D.G., Nauta, W.J.H.: Subcortical projections from the temporal neocortex in Macaca mulatta. J. Comp. Neurol. *106*, 183–212 (1956)

268. Wise, S.P.: The laminar organization of certain afferent and efferent fiber systems in the rat somatosensory cortex. Brain Res. *90*, 139–142 (1975)

269. Wise, S.P., Jones, E.G.: Cells of origin and terminal distribution of descending projections of the rat somatic sensory cortex. J. Comp. Neurol. *175*, 129–157 (1977)

270. Wong-Riley, M.T.T.: Demonstration of geniculo-cortical and callosal projection neurons in the squirrel monkey by means of retrograde axonal transport of horseradish peroxidase. Brain Res. *79*, 267–272 (1974)

271. Wyss, J.M.: Hypothalamic and brainstem afferents to the hippocampal formation in the rat. Neurosci. Abs. *3*, p. 209 (1977)

272. Wyss, J.M., Swanson, L.W., Cowan, W.M.: Species differences in the projection of Ammon's horn to the ipsilateral and contralateral dentate gyrus. Anat. Rec. *187*, 753 (1977)

Subject Index

In this index the first number (in Sans Serifs) refers to the figure; the second number corresponds to the number under which the pertinent structure can be found in the figure. Numbers following the abbreviation "p." refer to text-pages.

nucleus reticularis pontis caudalis, *syn: nucleus pontis centralis caudalis* 71.10; 112.9; 113.23; 131.11
nucleus reticularis pontis oralis, *syn: nucleus pontis centralis oralis* 70.7; 112.7; 113.20; 131.8
nucleus reticularis tegmenti pontis (Bechterew), *syn: nucleus papillioformis* 70.9; 71.14; 112.8; 119.7
nucleus reticularis thalami 35.18; 61.4; 125.9; 127.6; 152.6
nucleus retroambiguus 77.6
nucleus ruber 35.28; 114.2; 118.1; 119.3; 137.21; p. 154
nucleus ruber, pars magnocellularis 67.10; 120.8; 128.10
nucleus ruber, pars parvocellularis 65.12; 120.7; 128.9
nucleus sensorius principalis nervi trigemini 71.8; 99.7; 100.13
nucleus septi lateralis 146.6
nucleus septi medialis 141B.7
nucleus solitarius 75.4; 101.8; p. 119
nucleus solitarius, pars cardiorespiratoria 102.11
nucleus solitarius, pars gustatoria 102.9
nucleus spinalis nervi trigemini 99.8
nucleus spinalis nervi trigemini, pars caudalis 76.8–10; 100.17
nucleus spinalis nervi trigemini, pars interpolaris 75.8; 100.16
nucleus spinalis nervi trigemini, pars oralis 73.9; 100.15
nucleus subcuneiformis 112.6
nucleus subthalamicus, *syn: corpus subthalamicum (Luys)* 48.35; 61.10; 127.11; 128.8; 129.13; p. 170
nucleus suprachiasmaticus p. 131
nucleus supraopticus 58.9; 59.8; 135.13; 153.7
nucleus supraspinalis 77.8
nucleus tegmentalis dorsalis (Gudden) 101.3; 102.5; 137.24; 140.20; 154.20; p. 187
nucleus tegmentalis pedunculopontinus, pars compacta 69.9; 112.11
nucleus tegmentalis pedunculopontinus, pars dissipata 68.8
nucleus thoracicus, *syn: columna Clarki (Stilling-Clarke)* 86.5; 90.9; 115.23; p. 153
nucleus ventralis anterior 24.5; 60.5; 120.5; 121.6; 129.5
nucleus ventralis lateralis 24.9; 61.3; 120.4; 121.7; 129.4
nucleus ventralis posterior (nucleus ventralis posteroinferior, nucleus ventralis posterolateralis and nucleus ventralis posteromedialis) 121.8
nucleus ventralis posteroinferior 104.19
nucleus ventralis posterolateralis 24.6; 62.8; 95.2; 96.4; 98.3

nucleus ventralis posteromedialis 25.13; 62.11; 99.1+13; 100.3; 101.1
nucleus ventralis posteromedialis, pars parvocellularis 62.12; 102.3; 121.9
nucleus ventromedialis (hypothalami) 60.10; 135.9; 140.11; 141B.12
nucleus vestibularis inferior 73.5; 74.2; 103.7; 104.14
nucleus vestibularis lateralis (Deiters) 72.6; 73.3; 103.9; 104.23; p. 128
nucleus vestibularis medialis 72.7; 74.3; 103.6; 104.13
nucleus vestibularis superior 71.5; 72.5; 103.5; 104.9

Obex 14.15; 15.46
olfactory system p. 196
oliva (inferior), see also nucleus olivaris inferior 14.36; 17.35; p. 154
oliva superior (complex) p. 129
oliva superior, nucleus lateralis, *syn: nucleus lateralis olivae superioris* 72.14; 105.9; 106.9
oliva superior, nucleus medialis, *syn: nucleus medialis olivae superioris, nucleus accessorius olivae superioris* 72.15; 105.10; 106.10
operculum frontale 4.7; 8.10
operculum frontoparietale 4.5; 8.4
operculum temporale 4.6; 8.11

Pars intermedia cerebelli, see: hemisphaerium cerebelli, pars intermedia
pedunculus cerebellaris inferior, *syn: corpus restiforme* 18.5; 48.14; 74.18; 114.9; 117.13; p. 153
pedunculus cerebellaris medius, *syn: brachium pontis* 18.6; 49.16; 71.33; 114.10; 115.7; p. 153
pedunculus cerebellaris superior, *syn: brachium conjunctivum* 18.2; 47.10; 66.31; 118.9; 119.5; p. 153
pedunculus cerebellaris superior, ramus descendens 70.21; 115.3; 118.4; 119.6
pedunculus cerebri, *syn: crus cerebri* 14.21; 35.33; 42.29; 62.30; 126.13–15; p. 169
pedunculus corporis mamillaris 67.28; 134.14; 140.19; p. 189
pedunculus flocculi 18.22; 73.18
pedunculus nuclei lentiformis 28.12
pedunculus thalami anterior 48.28; 54.4; 58.22; 123.12; p. 163
pedunculus thalami inferior 123.14; 137.12; 143.3; p. 163
pedunculus thalami posterior 123.8; p. 163
pedunculus thalami superior 123.7; p. 163
pes hippocampi 34.42
plexus choroideus ventriculi lateralis 33.19; 35.32; 36.19; 52.9

A. Wackenheim

Radiodiagnosis of the Vertebrae in Adults

125 Exercises for Students and Practitioners
Exercises in Radiological Diagnosis
1983. 250 figures. VI, 176 pages
ISBN 3-540-11681-8

Designed for use both as an exercise manual for beginners
and as a refresher course for practitioners, the books in this
series aim toward the recognition and correct interpretation of
roentgenological signs. The authors deliberately omit clinical
or pathophysiological background information in the cases
presented in order to confront the reader directly with the lan-
guage of radio-imaging. The same didactic format is followed
for each of the body areas or organ systems covered: the
authors include normal and abnormal images as well as those
displaying pathognomic signs, evaluate their information level,
and discuss their significance in diagnosis.

Human Physiology

Editors: R. F. Schmidt, G. Thews
Translated from the German by M. A. Biederman-Thorson
1983. 569 figures (most in color). XXI, 725 pages
ISBN 3-540-11669-9

Fundamentals of Neurophysiology

Editor: R. F. Schmidt
With contributions by J. Dudel, W. Jänig, R. F. Schmidt,
M. Zimmermann
Translated from the German by M. A. Biederman-Thorson
Springer Study Edition
2nd revised and enlarged edition. 1978.
137 figures. IX, 339 pages
ISBN 3-540-08188-7

Fundamentals of Sensory Physiology

Editor: R. F. Schmidt
With contributions by H. Altner, J. Dudel, O.-J. Grüsser,
U. Grüsser-Cornehls, R. Klinke, R. F. Schmidt,
M. Zimmermann
Translated from the German by M. A. Biederman-Thorson
Springer Study Edition
2nd corrected edition. 1981. 139 figures. XI, 286 pages
ISBN 3-540-10349-X

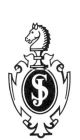

Springer-Verlag
Berlin
Heidelberg
New York
Tokyo

E. Braak
On the Structure of the Human Striate Area

1982. 44 figures. VI, 87 pages. (Advances in Anatomy, Embryology and Cell Biology, Volume 77)
ISBN 3-540-11512-9

A. G. Brown
Organization in the Spinal Cord

The Anatomy and Physiology of Identified Neurones

1981. 148 figures. XII, 238 pages
ISBN 3-540-10549-2

The Cranial Nerves

Anatomy · Pathology · Pathophysiology · Diagnosis · Treatment

Editors: M. Samii, P. J. Jannetta
1981. 410 figures. XVII, 664 pages
ISBN 3-540-10620-0

J. Lang
Clinical Anatomy of the Head

Neurocranium – Orbit – Craniocervical Regions

Translated from the German by R. R. Wilson, D. P. Winstanley
1982. 388 color photographs and 189 diagrams. XIV, 489 pages
ISBN 3-540-11014-3

Neural Coding of Motor Performance

Editors: J. Massion, J. Paillard, W. Schultz, M. Wiesendanger
1983. 88 figures, 7 tables. XI, 348 pages.
(Experimental Brain Research, Supplement 7)
ISBN 3-540-12140-4

Neuroradiology

A Neuropathological Approach

By R. Kautzky, K. J. Zülch. S. Wende, A. Tänzer
Translated from the German edition by W. M. Boehm
1982. 251 figures. XII, 324 pages
ISBN 3-540-10934-X

Positron Emission Tomography of the Brain

Editors: W.-D. Heiss, M. F. Phelps
1983. 98 figures. 300 pages
ISBN 3-540-12130-7

Techniques in Neuroanatomical Research

Editors: C. Heym, W.-G. Forssmann
1981. 165 figures. XIII, 395 pages
ISBN 3-540-10686-3

C. D. Woody
Memory, Learning and Higher Function

A Cellular View

1982. 134 figures. XIV, 483 pages
ISBN 3-540-90525-1

L. Záborszky
Afferent Connections of the Medial Basal Hypothalamus

1982. 31 figures. VIII, 107 pages.
(Advances in Anatomy, Embryology and Cell Biology, Volume 69)
ISBN 3-540-11076-3

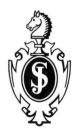

Springer-Verlag Berlin Heidelberg New York Tokyo